The Exotic Rice Hack Diet

Discover the World's Best-Kept Secrets for Weight Loss, 365 Days of Delicious Recipes to Transform Your Diet with Global Rice Varieties

Access your FREE bonus Guide!

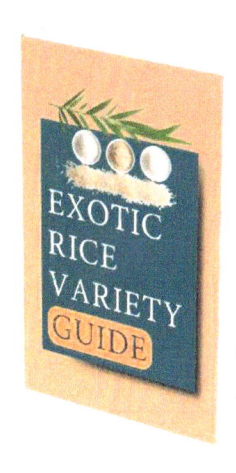

As a valued reader of "The Exotic Rice Hack Diet," we're excited to offer you an exclusive gift: **The Exotic Rice Variety Guide**—absolutely free!

This comprehensive guide is your passport to discovering the world's most flavorful and nutritious rice varieties. Elevate your meals, explore new cultures, and embark on a global culinary adventure—all from the comfort of your kitchen.

Scan the QR code to Grab your copy!

Table of Contents

INTRODUCTION _____ 5

CHAPTER 1: THE RICE ADVANTAGE _____ 6
  Rice Rehab: Why It's NOT the Enemy _____ 7
  Nutrient Powerhouse: What's Inside Every Grain _____ 9
  Fullness = Satisfaction: _____ 11
  How Rice Conquers Cravings _____ 11
  Portion Perfection: _____ 12
  Mindful Eating with Rice _____ 12

CHAPTER 2: EXOTIC RICE REVOLUTION _____ 14
  Around the World in 80 Grains: Explore the Rice Universe _____ 16
  Flavor Explosion: Taste the Difference _____ 17

CHAPTER 3: IS THE RICE HACK RIGHT FOR YOU? _____ 19
  (Almost) Everyone Benefits: Why This Plan Works. _____ 20
  Gluten-Free Goodness: Your Natural Choice _____ 21
  Adaptable Feasting: Your Diet, Your Way _____ 23

CHAPTER 4: RISE & SHINE BREAKFASTS _____ 25

CHAPTER 5: LUNCHTIME LEGENDS _____ 39

CHAPTER 6: SPEEDY & SATISFYING SNACKS _____ 50

CHAPTER 7: DINNER DELIGHTS _____ 62

INDEX OF RECIPES _____ 73

INTRODUCTION

Picture this: It's Monday morning, and you're staring at the scale in despair. Another weekend of takeout and "treating yourself" has left you feeling sluggish and further from your weight loss goals. Diets in the past? They've involved endless salads, tasteless grilled chicken, and a constant battle against cravings. Sure, you'd lose a few pounds...only to binge and regain them as soon as those bland meals became too much.

I know that struggle because I've lived it. Years of yo-yo dieting left me frustrated and believing that healthy eating was synonymous with boring food. But then, a trip to Southeast Asia changed everything. The bustling markets of Thailand, fragrant with spices, offered a revelation: rice. Not as a side dish, but as the star of the most vibrant and satisfying meals I'd ever tasted. From fluffy jasmine rice paired with fiery curries to nutty red rice in sweet-and-sour salads, I discovered a whole world of flavor I never knew existed.

The best part? I wasn't starving. I was energized, inspired, and those extra pounds started to melt away without the usual deprivation. Back home, I made it my mission to harness the power of rice on my own health journey. The Exotic Rice Hack was born.

This isn't some restrictive fad diet. It's a delicious lifestyle shift, an invitation to explore the incredible diversity the world of rice offers. Get ready to say goodbye to bland diet food and hello to:

- Crispy Persian rice studded with tart barberries and pistachios
- Spanish-inspired paella brimming with fresh seafood and smoky spices
- Creamy coconut rice pudding infused with warm spices and tropical mango

Imagine shedding those extra pounds without constantly feeling hungry or deprived. That's the power of the Exotic Rice Hack. Rice is incredibly satisfying and provides your body with balanced energy – no more cravings sabotaging your progress! Plus, you'll wave goodbye to that afternoon slump. The fiber in rice supports healthy digestion and steady blood sugar levels, powering you with feel-good energy that lasts. But the best part? This plan is a delicious journey. Each meal becomes an opportunity to explore vibrant flavors, textures, and cuisines from around the globe. Forget boring diet food – this is about celebrating the endless possibilities that rice offers.

However, let's be clear: the Exotic Rice Hack isn't a magic, overnight solution. It's about changing your relationship with food, one delicious grain at a time. By embracing sustainable shifts and nourishing your body with real, satisfying meals, you'll achieve lasting results and a newfound appreciation for healthy eating.

Adventure awaits! With the Exotic Rice Hack Diet, you'll discover how to lose weight, feel your best, and cultivate a joyful relationship with food. Let's transform your plate, one delicious grain at a time!

Chapter 1:
The Rice Advantage

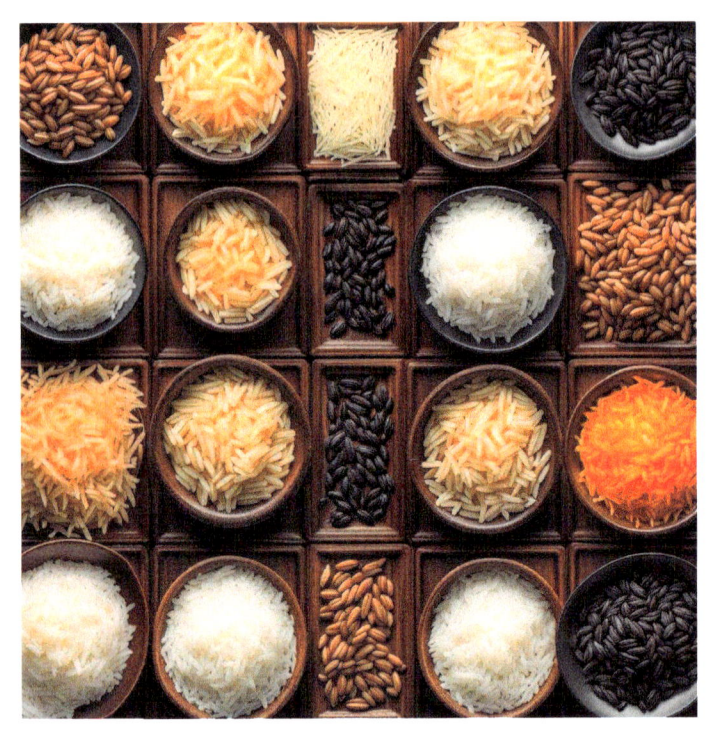

For years, rice has been the victim of bad press. It's blamed for weight gain, dismissed as "empty carbs," and relegated to a forgettable side dish. But let's take a step back for a moment. Venture with me, in your mind's eye, to bustling street markets in Thailand, fragrant with lemongrass and sizzling spices. Or perhaps a traditional Japanese home, where a steaming bowl of perfectly cooked rice is the centerpiece of a nourishing meal. In countless cultures across the globe, rice isn't merely food; it's woven into the fabric of daily life, a symbol of sustenance and tradition.

So, how can something so deeply cherished, so fundamentally nourishing, be simultaneously painted as the enemy of our waistlines in Western diet culture? The truth is, rice itself isn't inherently "bad." It's often what we do to it, how we portion it, and the overwhelmingly processed world of food we pair it with that leads to problems.

It's time to bust those myths, clear away the misconceptions, and rediscover the incredible potential this humble grain holds. Get ready to question everything you think you know about rice. It might just transform your health, revitalize your meals, and unlock a newfound joy of eating. Are you ready to open your mind – and your kitchen – to the world of possibilities that rice offers?

Rice Rehab:
Why It's NOT The Enemy

For starters, we need to address the elephant in the room: calories. Yes, rice, like any food, contains calories. A cup of cooked brown rice provides roughly 216 calories, placing it in the same ballpark as other whole-grain staples like quinoa (222 calories per cup) or whole-wheat pasta (220 calories per cup). However, calories are just one piece of the puzzle. The Okinawa Diet, a dietary pattern linked to exceptional longevity in Japan, centers around white rice as a major source of carbohydrates. This seemingly contradictory fact highlights a crucial concept: it's not just the type of rice, but how it fits into your overall dietary picture.

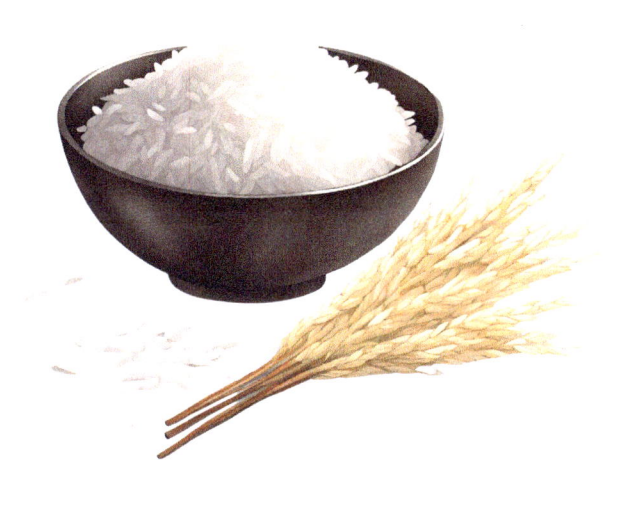

Weight gain is a complex issue influenced by numerous factors beyond simply "calories in, calories out." Studies published in the American Journal of Clinical Nutrition (2010) found no significant difference in weight loss between participants who consumed moderate portions of white rice compared to those who ate other carbohydrate sources. The key lies in portion control and creating balanced meals. A plate overflowing with white rice and minimal vegetables won't do your health any favors. However, when incorporated strategically as part of a meal rich in lean protein, colorful vegetables, and healthy fats (think avocado or olive oil), rice becomes a valuable tool for supporting weight loss goals.

Let's unpack the Glycemic Index (GI). This index ranks carbohydrates based on how quickly they raise blood sugar levels. White rice does have a higher GI than, say, brown rice (73 for white rice vs. 50 for brown rice). This means white rice can cause a faster blood sugar spike. However, a 2020 research review published in the journal Nutrients emphasizes that GI is just one factor influencing blood sugar response. Here's the good news: how rice is cooked plays a role. Studies from the International Journal of Food Science & Technology (2016) indicate that cooking rice using techniques like the "absorption method" (limited water, cooked until all water is absorbed) leads to a lower GI compared to methods with excess water.

WHAT YOU PAIR WITH RICE

significantly impacts blood sugar response. Including protein sources like grilled salmon or skinless chicken alongside rice helps slow down digestion and sugar absorption. Fiber-rich vegetables like broccoli or carrots add another layer of control, while healthy fats from avocado or olive oil further contribute to a balanced blood sugar response.

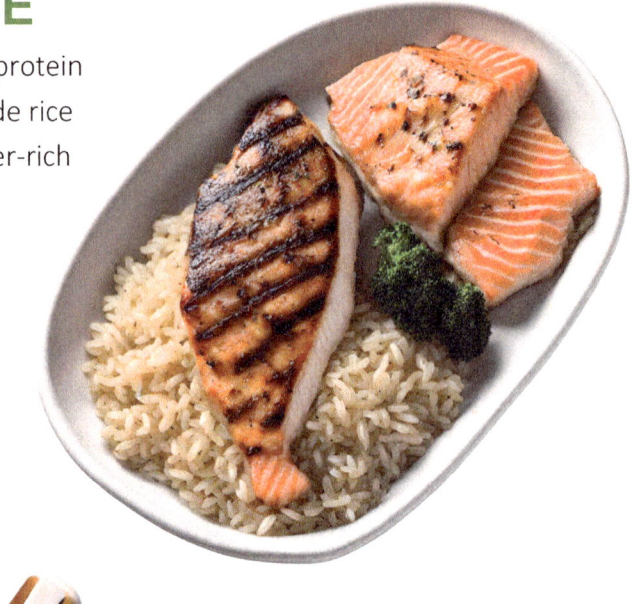

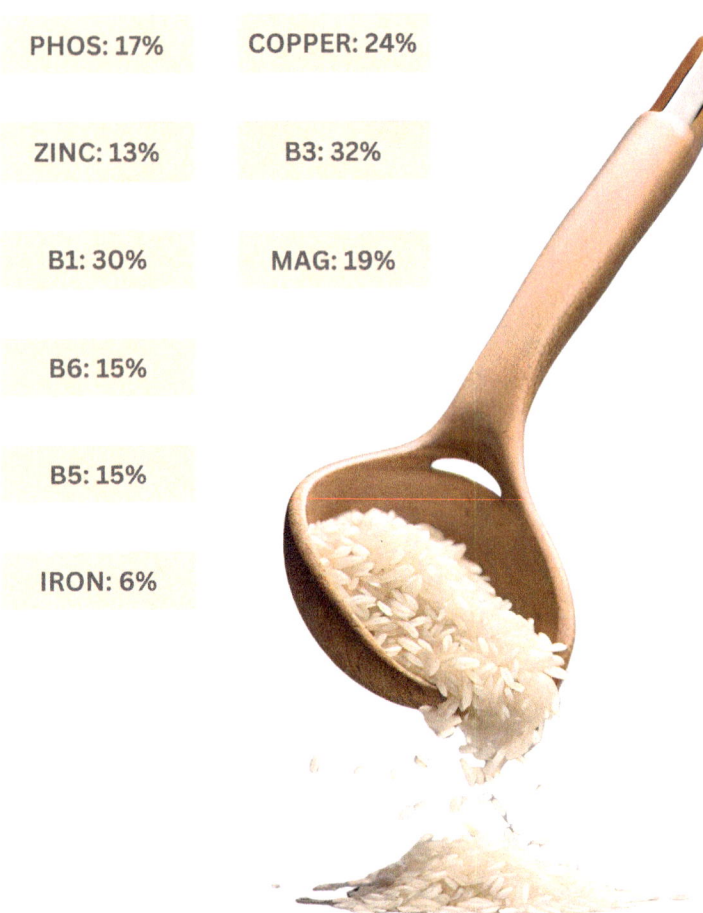

PHOS: 17%
COPPER: 24%
ZINC: 13%
B3: 32%
B1: 30%
MAG: 19%
B6: 15%
B5: 15%
IRON: 6%

When it comes to rice varieties, we have a spectrum of nutritional powerhouses to choose from. Brown rice reigns supreme, boasting a wealth of fiber (3.5 grams per cup), magnesium (84 mg per cup), and B vitamins like thiamin and niacin, crucial for energy production. Red rice, cultivated in places like the Himalayan foothills, is an antioxidant powerhouse, containing compounds like anthocyanins that may offer heart-protective benefits. Black rice, often referred to as "forbidden rice" due to its historical rarity in China, boasts a unique black hull rich in anthocyanins and fiber. However, let's not dismiss white rice entirely. Enriched white rice offers readily available iron, essential for oxygen transport in the body, and certain B vitamins that play a role in nerve function and cell metabolism.

The true culprit might be hiding in plain sight on your grocery store shelves: those tempting "rice products" marketed as healthy alternatives. Rice cakes, crackers, and puffed cereals often lack the fiber-rich bran layer present in whole grain rice. This not only reduces their nutritional value but also diminishes their ability to keep you feeling satisfied. The refined nature of these products combined with potential added sugars can lead to overeating and negate any perceived health benefits.

The bottom line: whole grain rice, enjoyed in sensible portions as part of a balanced diet, can be a fantastic ally for weight loss and overall health. Explore the colorful world of rice varieties, experiment with cooking techniques, and pair your rice dishes with a symphony of nutritious ingredients. You might be surprised at how delicious and supportive this versatile grain can be on your wellness journey.

Nutrient Powerhouse:
What's Inside Every Grain

Rice delivers energy to your body primarily through complex carbohydrates. Unlike the simple sugars found in soda or processed sweets, complex carbs break down gradually. This translates to an extended release of glucose into your bloodstream, fueling your cells in a sustained manner. Picture the difference between the short-lived rush from a chocolate bar versus the steady, focused energy rice provides – that's the power of complex carbohydrates in action! This balanced energy delivery system is key to feeling satiated, reducing those pesky mid-afternoon cravings that can sabotage weight loss efforts.

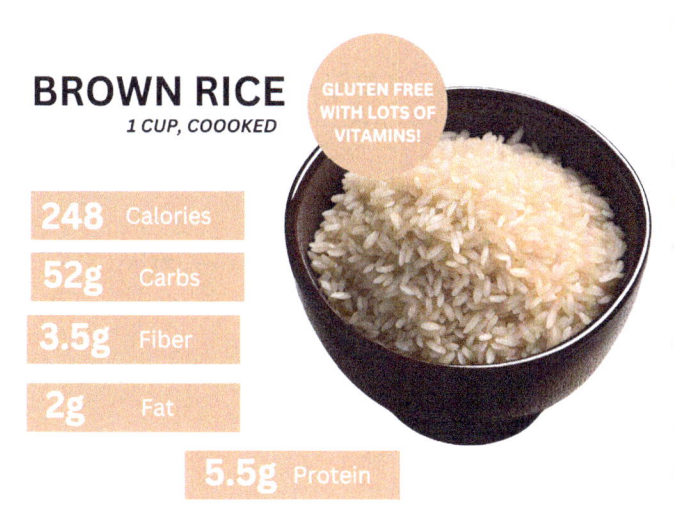

BROWN RICE
1 CUP, COOOKED

GLUTEN FREE WITH LOTS OF VITAMINS!

- 248 Calories
- 52g Carbs
- 3.5g Fiber
- 2g Fat
- 5.5g Protein

While not a protein superstar like beans or chicken breast, rice does contribute modestly to your daily protein needs. A cup of cooked brown rice contains roughly 5.5 grams of protein, while white rice contains around 4 grams per cup. Remember, every little bit adds up! Combined with other protein-rich foods throughout the day, rice supports muscle maintenance and repair, crucial for both fitness goals and overall vitality.

Let's talk micronutrients – the mighty vitamins and minerals where rice, especially brown rice, truly excels. Brown rice is packed with B-vitamins, including thiamin (B1), riboflavin (B2), niacin (B3), and pyridoxine (B6). These B-vitamins act as tiny powerhouses within your cells, facilitating the conversion of food into energy to combat fatigue and keep your metabolism humming. Brown rice also offers a solid dose of magnesium, approximately 84 milligrams per cup. Magnesium is essential for hundreds of processes within your body, including healthy blood pressure regulation, nerve function, and bone health. Another mineral found in brown rice is manganese (1.8 milligrams per cup), a vital component of antioxidant systems that defends your cells against damage and supports immune function.

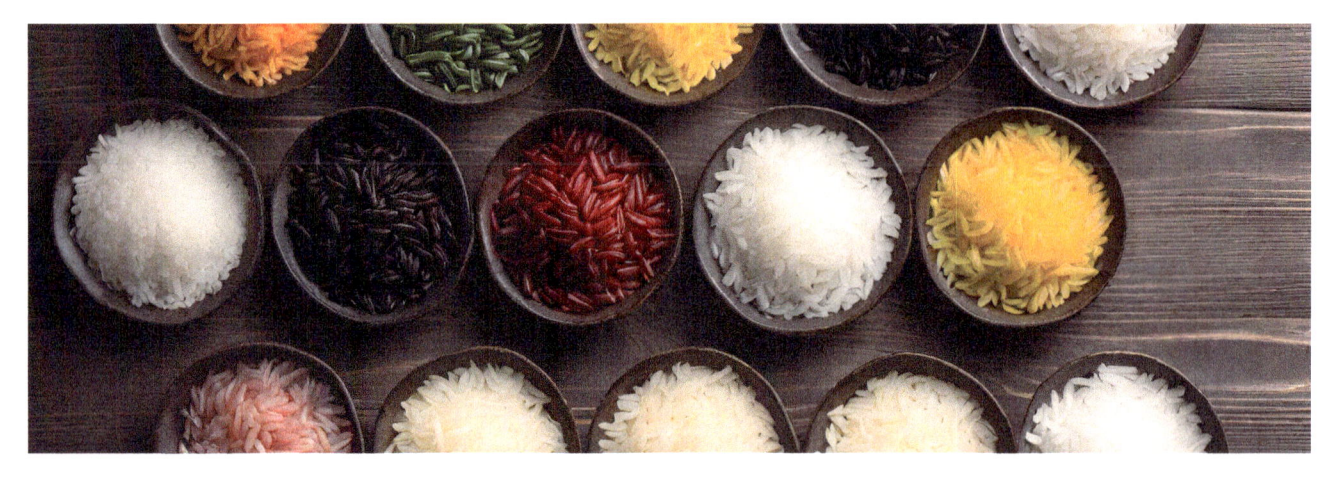

The vibrant colors of rice varieties like red or black rice reveal the presence of potent antioxidants called anthocyanins. These compounds have been studied for their potential to protect heart health by reducing inflammation and may even offer protective effects against age-related cognitive decline, as suggested by a 2016 review published in the journal Nutrients.

Finally, let's get into resistant starch, a fascinating type of carbohydrate. Think of resistant starch as a special type of fiber that, as its name suggests, resists digestion in your small intestine. Interestingly, cooking rice and then cooling it actually increases its resistant starch content. Studies suggest this resistant starch functions as a prebiotic, fueling the beneficial bacteria in your gut. A thriving gut microbiome can positively impact digestive health, and interestingly enough, may even offer indirect benefits for weight management and immune health.

See? The humble grain of rice becomes a complex and fascinating nutritional powerhouse when we look a bit closer. It's a source of sustained energy, key vitamins and minerals, and even unique compounds that promote a healthy gut. All this makes rice a smart and delicious addition to your weight loss plan!

Fullness = Satisfaction:
How Rice Conquers Cravings

The key player in this satiety story is fiber. Unlike refined, processed carbohydrates that are rapidly digested, the fiber in rice, especially whole grain varieties, adds significant bulk to your meals. This isn't just about feeling full for a few minutes; it's about triggering a cascade of signals that tell your body you've had enough to eat.

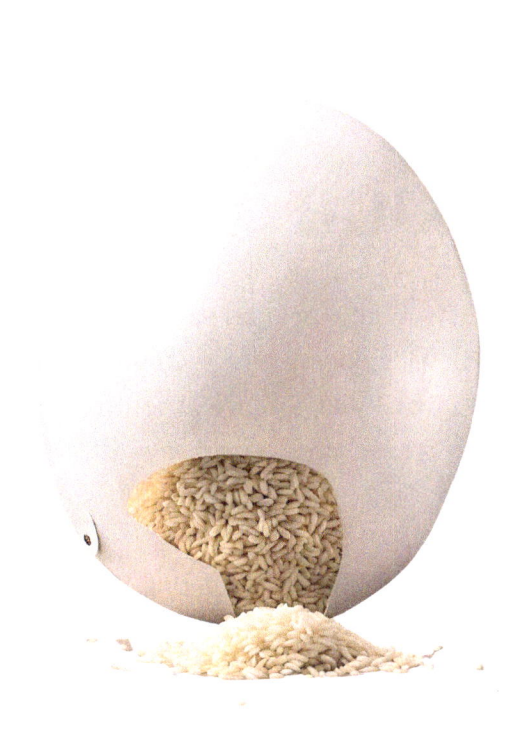

Picture your stomach as a balloon. When you eat fiber-rich foods, that balloon gently expands, stretching specialized receptors within the stomach lining. These receptors send signals via the vagus nerve (a major player in the gut-brain axis) to your brain, essentially saying, "Hey up there, we're getting full down here!" A 2017 study published in the journal Nutrition Reviews highlighted the role of insoluble fiber, found in abundance in brown rice, in stimulating the release of specific hormones like peptide YY, which play a role in suppressing appetite and promoting satiety.

Fiber also puts the brakes on digestion. Unlike a candy bar that's absorbed with alarming speed, fiber slows the passage of food through your digestive tract. This means your stomach empties at a more gradual pace, translating into prolonged feelings of fullness and reduced likelihood of those dreaded hunger pangs striking prematurely throughout the day.

Let's not forget the remarkable ability of rice to interact with liquids. During cooking, each grain acts like a tiny sponge, absorbing a significant amount of water and physically expanding in volume. This expansion takes up valuable real estate in your stomach, amplifying the fullness factor. For instance, just a half cup of uncooked brown rice can yield approximately two cups of cooked rice, creating a satisfying portion that can help you feel full.

While a bowl of perfectly cooked brown rice is satisfying on its own, for the ultimate hunger-busting meal, think of rice as a brilliant foundation. Pairing it with lean proteins like grilled fish, lentils, or black beans delivers essential amino acids, the building blocks of protein that further contribute to feelings of satiety. A generous portion of fiber-packed vegetables like spinach sauteed with garlic, roasted Brussels sprouts, or a rainbow bell pepper salad adds even more bulk and an irresistible array of textures, keeping your meal interesting and enjoyable. This strategic pairing of rice, protein, and vegetables is supported by research from the journal 'Appetite' (2016), emphasizing the combined power of fiber and protein to reduce hunger and keep you feeling full for longer.

Rice's ability to combat cravings isn't just theoretical; it's also supported by traditional dietary patterns. Many Asian cuisines, known for their emphasis on rice-based dishes, often enjoy lower rates of obesity compared to those following predominantly Western dietary patterns.

So, the next time you crave a satisfying, hunger-busting meal, turn to the power of rice. Let those fluffy grains, bursting with fiber, become your secret weapon in the battle against cravings. Combine them with vibrant vegetables and lean protein sources for a complete and delicious approach to sustainable weight loss.

Portion Perfection:
Mindful Eating with Rice

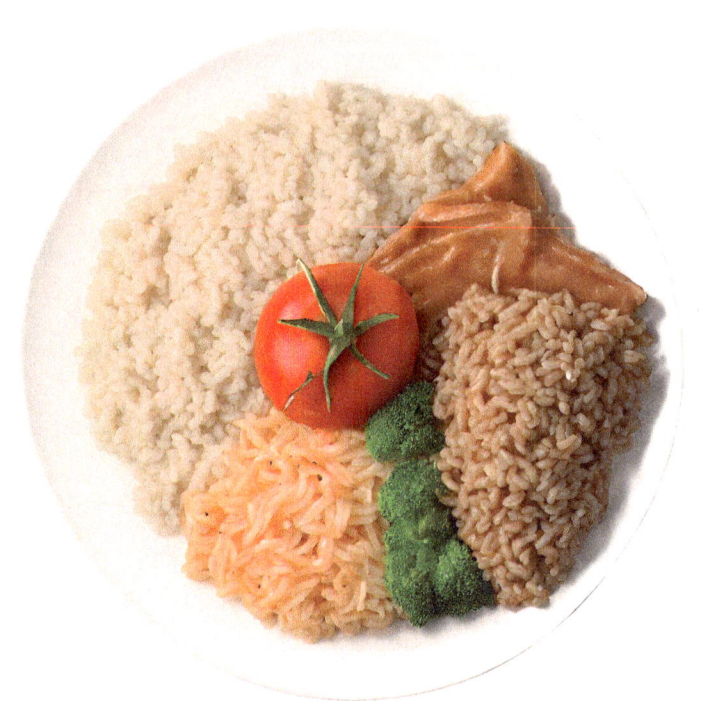

Weight loss isn't just about what you eat; it's about how you eat. By slowing down and truly tuning into your body's signals, you'll gain a sense of control over your food choices that goes far beyond any restrictive diet.

Start by setting the stage for mindful eating. Eliminate distractions – turn off the TV, put your phone away, and settle into a calm space. With each bite, pay close attention to the sensory experience. Is it slightly nutty brown rice, fluffy and fragrant basmati, or perhaps earthy wild rice with a hint of smokiness? Appreciate how the flavors mingle with other elements of your dish, the sweetness of roasted sweet potatoes, or the zesty burst of lemon on grilled fish.

The simple act of putting your fork down between bites provides a powerful interruption to mindless eating. This brief pause gives your digestive system precious time to send signals to your brain. Studies like the one published in the American Journal of Clinical Nutrition (2014) suggest that eating at a slower pace can promote fullness and potentially even decrease calorie intake. As you eat, check in with yourself periodically. Notice the sensations in your stomach, the gradual fading of hunger. Differentiate between feeling content and satiated, and that uncomfortable, overly-full sensation. Our aim is to stop before we reach that last point, leaving our bodies feeling nourished and energized.

To visualize portion control without resorting to scales and measuring cups, let's use the time-tested "plate method." Imagine your plate divided into quarters. One quarter is reserved for your rice, your satisfying carbohydrate base. Another quarter is dedicated to lean protein sources, such as grilled salmon, tofu, or a poached egg. The remaining half – yes, a full half of your plate – is where those vibrant vegetables shine! This strategic distribution helps you visualize the ideal balance of nutrients to support fullness, steady energy levels, and overall health.

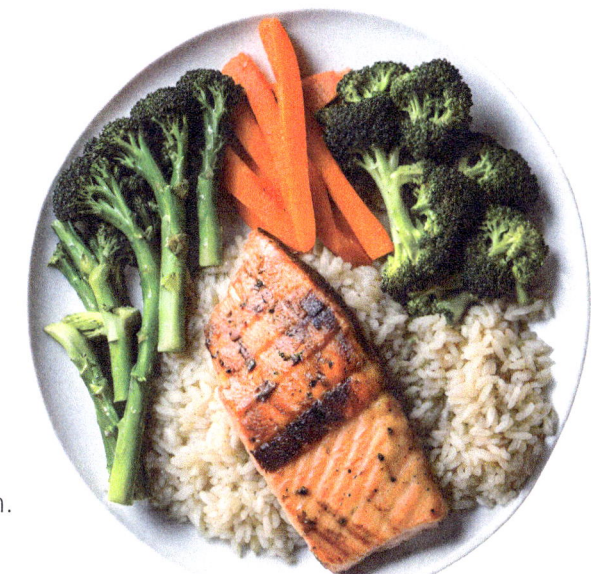

Mindful eating isn't about perfection. It's a journey of self-discovery, of cultivating a healthier, more intuitive relationship with food. Be patient with yourself, and remember, some days will be easier than others. The simple act of choosing rice is already a step towards nourishing your body with a satisfying whole food that supports your weight loss goals. Embrace the process, enjoy the flavors, and let mindful eating become a path to a happier, healthier you.

So often, we think about weight loss in terms of restriction and sacrifice. But with rice, the path to your goals can be both delicious and satisfying! You've learned how rice isn't the enemy, but a powerful tool. It's a source of steady energy, a natural appetite suppressant, and the foundation for countless nourishing and vibrant meals.

You now have the tools to approach portion sizes with confidence and cultivate mindful eating habits that will serve you long after the last grain of rice is gone. This isn't just about transforming your plate; it's about transforming your relationship with food. So, let's ditch the fad diets and embrace the power of real, unprocessed ingredients. It's time to fuel your body with joy, one delicious spoonful of rice at a time.

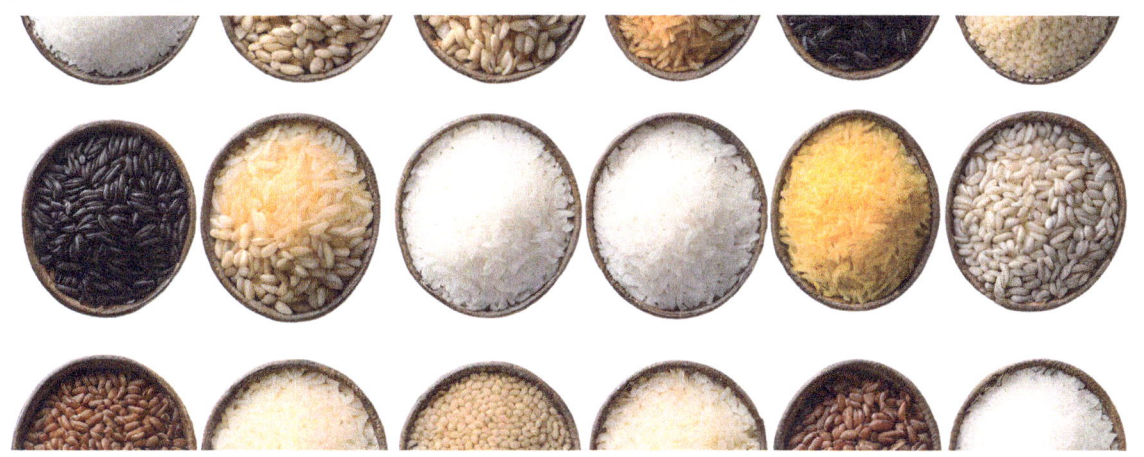

Chapter 2:
Exotic Rice Revolution

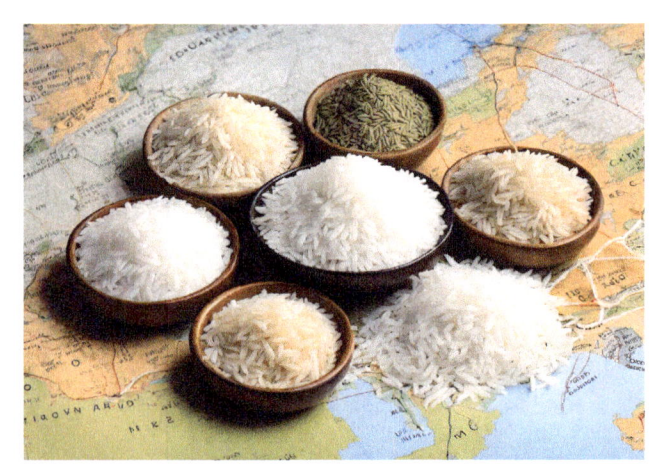

Think of your pantry as a portal to culinary adventures. For many of us, when it comes to rice, that portal has remained mostly closed. Sure, there's likely a bag of long-grain white rice, perhaps a box of brown for those extra healthy days. But the truth is, we're missing out on a world of flavors, textures, and surprisingly diverse nutritional profiles hidden within the vast and vibrant kingdom of rice.

Imagine unlocking a delicious secret, one that allows you to "travel" the globe without leaving your kitchen. From the fragrant fields of Thailand to the ancient terraces of the Himalayas, a simple switch of your rice can transport your tastebuds to exotic lands. Each variety boasts unique flavors and properties, offering exciting culinary possibilities while simultaneously enhancing your diet's nutritional value.

Let's start with a classic, white rice. While often dismissed as nutritionally inferior, it serves as a perfect blank canvas. Its delicate flavor effortlessly absorbs the bold spices of an Indian curry, the fresh herbs of a Mediterranean salad, or the smoky richness of Mexican cuisine. Enriched varieties offer a boost of iron and B vitamins, supporting energy production and overall well-being.

But why stop there? A whole universe of rice awaits! Journey to Thailand and discover the floral aroma of Jasmine rice, its soft, slightly sticky grains ideal for soaking up the vibrant flavors of a Thai green curry or stir-fry. From the foothills of the Himalayas comes Bhutanese Red Rice, a nutty, earthy grain packed with fiber and antioxidants. This rice makes a stunning addition to salads, its vibrant color adding a visual pop and nutritional punch.

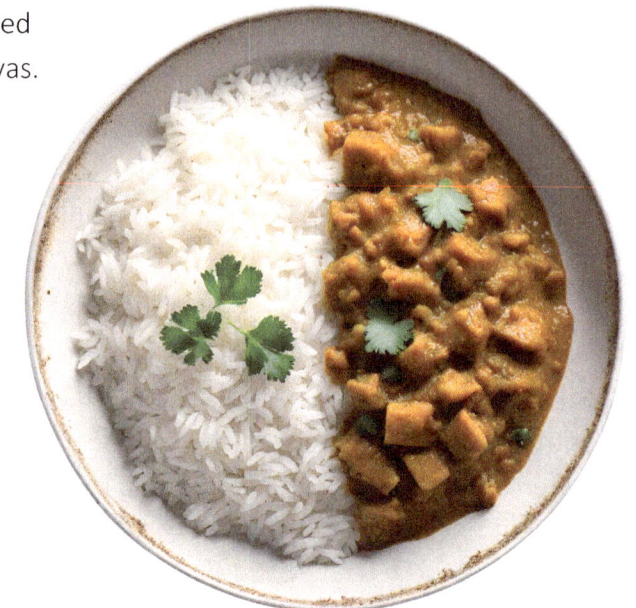

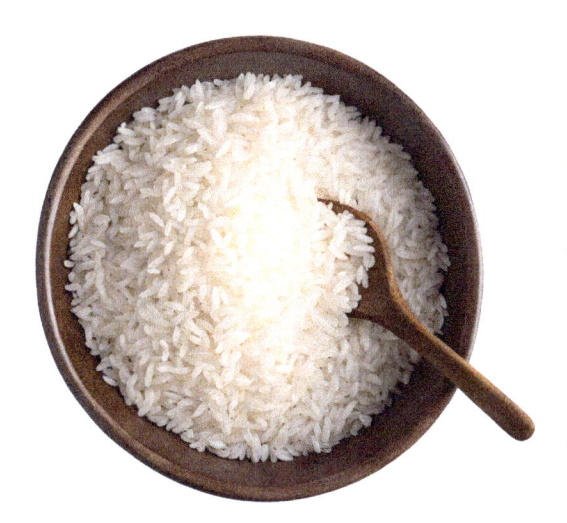

Venturing to Italy, we encounter Arborio rice, the creamy, plump-grained secret behind authentic risotto. As it cooks, Arborio releases starches, creating an irresistibly rich and satisfying dish bursting with flavor. Even wild rice, hailing from the lakes and wetlands of North America, offers a distinctly chewy texture and slightly smoky taste. It makes a satisfying alternative to ordinary rice, adding depth and complexity to soups, stews, or even as a base for unique grain bowls.

The benefits of exploring these exotic rice varieties extend far beyond taste. Each type offers its own nutritional gifts. Black rice, also known as 'forbidden rice' due to its historical exclusivity in ancient China, delivers a striking purplish-black hue thanks to potent antioxidants called anthocyanins. These same antioxidants are found in blueberries and have been researched for their potential benefits in protecting heart health and cognitive function.

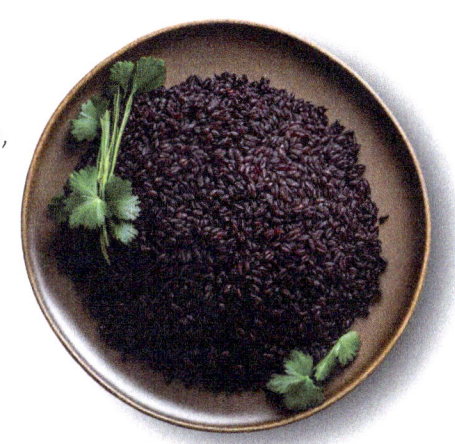

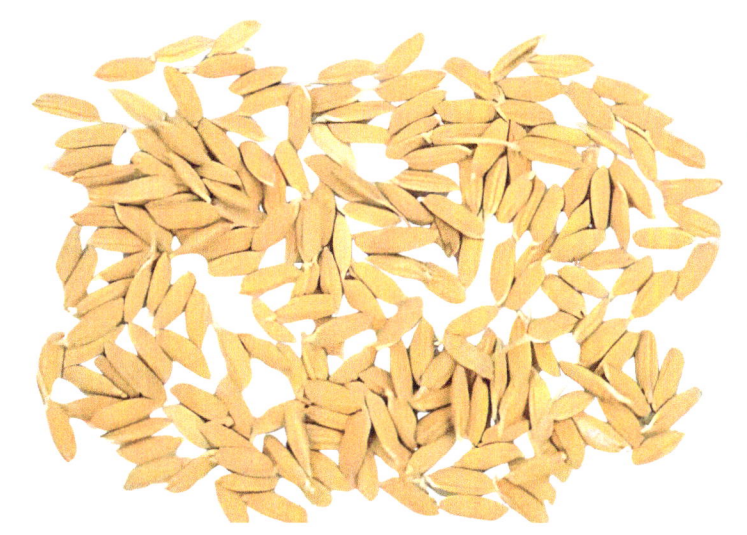

By diversifying your rice choices, you not only transform the familiar into the exciting but also become a conscious participant in a global food system. Sourcing heritage rice varieties like Carolina Gold, a prized grain with a storied history in the American South, or Wehani, a flavorful basmati-style rice developed in California, supports small-scale farmers and promotes agricultural biodiversity.

Choosing heirloom rice varieties not only benefits local economies but often supports more sustainable growing practices. Many traditional rice farms utilize natural methods that conserve water resources and minimize environmental impact. Exploring fair-trade options ensures that the farmers behind these unique grains receive equitable compensation for their labor.

Embracing the Exotic Rice Revolution is an invitation to step outside your culinary comfort zone and into a world of delicious possibilities. With each spoonful, you'll discover new flavors and textures, nourish your body with a wide array of nutrients, and even contribute to a better, more sustainable food system. So, let's ditch the "same old rice" routine and spice up our plates and lives with the vibrant diversity the rice world has to offer. Let the flavors transport you, the textures delight you, and the journey of exploration awaken a newfound appreciation for this humble yet incredibly versatile grain!

Around the World in 80 Grains:
Explore the Rice Universe

Picture yourself traversing the foothills of the mighty Himalayas, where the unique terroir gives rise to Bhutanese Red Rice. Nestled amidst terraced paddies, this ancient grain thrives at high altitudes, developing a distinctive nutty flavor, chewy texture, and eye-catching reddish-brown hue. Packed with fiber and antioxidants, it's a culinary treasure and a testament to the ingenuity of Himalayan farmers.

A hop over to Southeast Asia takes us to the lush, sun-drenched paddies of Thailand, where the fragrant fields are alive with the cultivation of Jasmine rice. Each grain carries a delicate floral aroma, a signature of this beloved long-grain variety. Jasmine rice, with its soft, slightly sticky texture, has a remarkable ability to absorb the vibrant flavors of Thai cuisine, from fiery curries to the fresh, zesty notes of herbs and lemongrass.

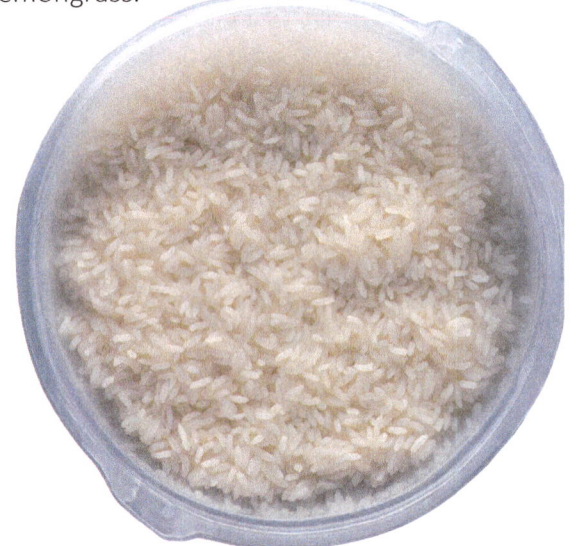

Speaking of sticky textures, no rice adventure would be complete without venturing into the realm of short-grain glutinous rice. Known as "sweet rice" in many Asian cultures, this unique type transforms when cooked, becoming delightfully soft, chewy, and slightly sweet. From the bustling streets of Tokyo, where it's skillfully molded into perfect sushi, to the vibrant markets of Bangkok, where it forms the base of the iconic dessert Mango Sticky Rice, glutinous rice demonstrates that rice can be both savory and sweet.

The journey continues with the intriguing Forbidden Rice, also known as black rice. Once reserved for emperors in ancient China, it's gaining popularity globally. Its striking purplish-black hue comes from anthocyanins, the same potent antioxidants found in blueberries. Studies from the journal Nutrients (2020) suggest that black rice may play a role in protecting heart health and reducing inflammation. And how about those subtly smoky, earthy notes of North American wild rice? Prized for its chewy texture and nutritional density, this grain, hailing from the lakes of Minnesota and Canada, adds a distinctive touch to grain bowls, soups, and beyond.

The Exotic Rice Revolution isn't just about tantalizing your taste buds; it's about connecting with the cultural heritage, agricultural ingenuity, and nutritional diversity hidden within each and every grain. Get ready to discover recipes that showcase these unique varieties and unlock a whole new world of culinary possibilities!

Flavor Explosion:
Taste the Difference

It's time to dismantle the myth of bland rice and embark on a scientific exploration of flavor! Forget about tasteless side dishes; every type of rice boasts a unique profile of subtle aromas and tastes waiting to be discovered. Think of this flavor discovery as an experiment for your senses, where you'll learn that rice can be nutty, earthy, subtly sweet, or even carry delicate floral notes.

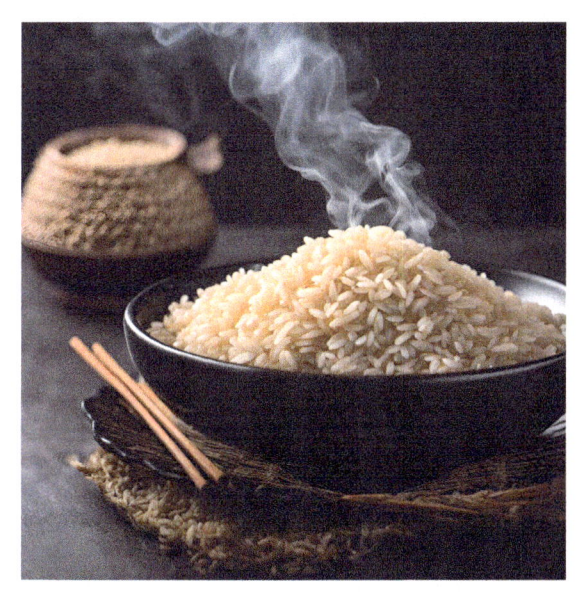

Let's start by challenging your preconceived notions. Next time you make a pot of brown rice, take a moment, inhale its aroma, and then actively taste it. Do you notice a delicate nutty flavor, perhaps a gentle toastiness? This inherent flavor of brown rice is due to naturally occuring compounds that become more pronounced with cooking. Now try wild rice. Often harvested from the lakes of Minnesota and Canada, wild rice delivers an earthy note with a subtle, delicious smokiness that reflects its unique habitat and traditional processing techniques. And of course, no exploration of rice would be complete without basmati, this iconic variety grown in the foothills of the Himalayas, loved for its intoxicating floral fragrance.

Your nose is a powerful tool on this journey of discovery! As basmati rice cooks, it releases a tantalizing aroma reminiscent of popcorn – this unique scent profile is due to the presence of a compound called 2-Acetyl-1-pyrroline. For an earthy experience, cook up some Bhutanese Red Rice. Its subtle aroma offers a hint of its ancient origins and the high-altitude Himalayan environment where it thrives.

Now here's where the fun truly begins: flavor infusions! Elevate your favorite rice with simple additions during the cooking process. Adding a single bay leaf to your pot of basmati creates a subtle but delightful shift in flavor. For a warming, cozy twist, try adding a whole cinnamon stick to your brown rice. The gentle cinnamon flavor perfectly complements the inherent nuttiness of the rice, especially in dishes with Mexican or Middle Eastern influences.

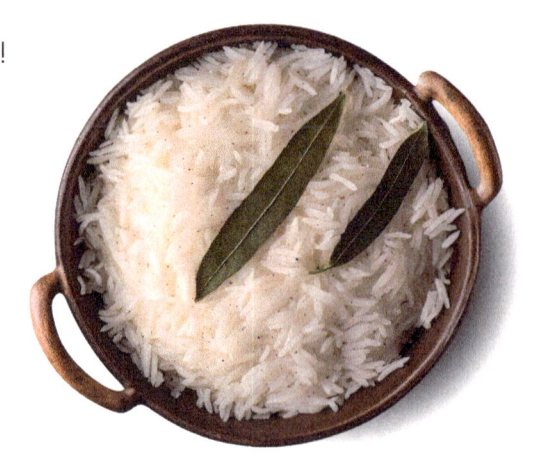

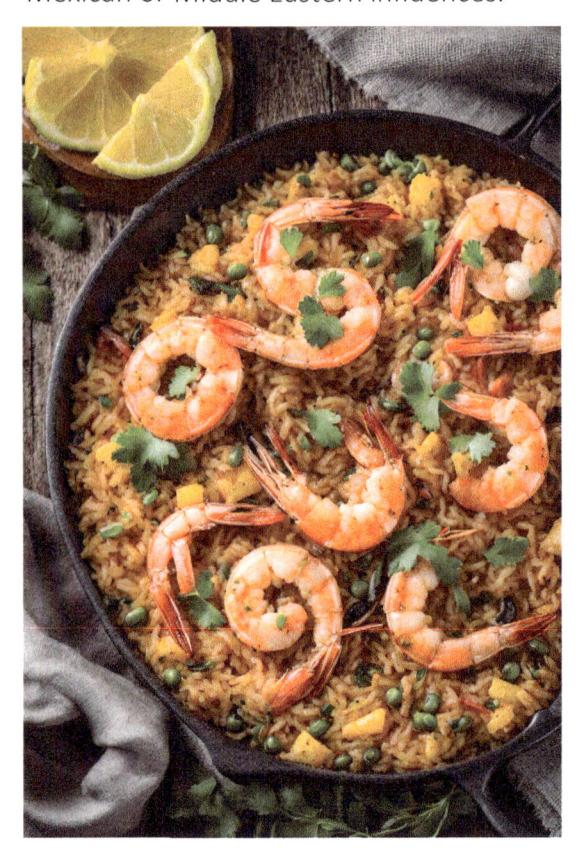

Certain types of rice could be crowned champions of flavor absorption. Spanish Bomba rice, the secret to an authentic, flavorful paella, takes on the rich flavors of saffron, spices, and seafood broth while maintaining its structural integrity. Similarly, Italian Arborio rice, famed for its role in risotto, gradually releases starches during cooking. This creates the characteristic creamy texture while allowing the rice to soak up flavors, transforming a simple dish into a luxurious celebration of taste.

The days of rice being labeled as "boring" are officially over! Your culinary adventure into the world of exotic rice has awakened your palate to the subtle flavors, intriguing aromas, and textures unique to each variety. It's clear that rice isn't merely a blank canvas; it's an active participant, capable of enhancing the overall taste of a dish.

With your newfound appreciation, you're no longer just cooking rice; you're embarking on a journey of sensory exploration with every pot. The next time you're in the rice aisle at the grocery store, let curiosity guide you. Reach for those intriguing bags of Bhutanese Red Rice, fragrant Jasmine, or perhaps a jar of wild rice.

This newfound appreciation for the symphony of flavors that different rice varieties offer will revolutionize the way you experience your meals. Each bite becomes an opportunity for discovery, showcasing a delightful interplay between the subtle nuances of the rice and the bold flavors of the dish it complements.

Chapter 3:
Is the Rice Hack Right for You?

Going on board on any nutritional change requires taking an honest look at where you're starting and the goals you have in mind. Finding a diet that's both effective and actually enjoyable is crucial. That's where the Exotic Rice Hack comes in. This way of eating centers around a versatile, satisfying whole food: rice. But it's not about rigid rules or miserable deprivation. Think of it as a delicious invitation to create a healthy relationship with food, one that fuels your body, satisfies your tastebuds, and leaves you feeling energized, not imprisoned by restrictive diets.

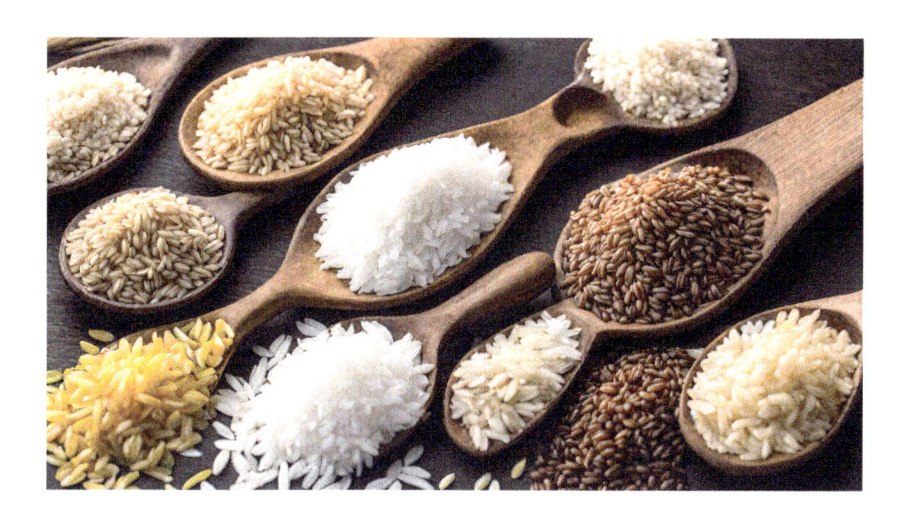

The beauty of rice lies in its adaptability. It welcomes a wide range of flavors and fits seamlessly into countless cuisines. This makes it a remarkably accessible starting point for those seeking to improve their diet without feeling a sense of deprivation.

While this plan offers structure and inspiration, it's truly about finding what works for YOU. Everyone has different needs, preferences, and lifestyles. Personalization is key! If you're someone who enjoys bold spices and the excitement of vibrant flavors, let those aromatic curries and stir-fries become your go-to. Or perhaps, the cozy comfort of a fragrant risotto resonates more with your palate. This journey encourages you to explore the world of rice and discover what makes you feel fueled, satisfied, and truly nourished.

The benefits of the Exotic Rice Hack extend far beyond weight loss. By prioritizing whole grains, plentiful vegetables, and lean proteins, you're not just transforming your plate, but potentially your overall well-being. Expect improved energy levels, better digestion, and perhaps most importantly, a newfound sense of freedom. Let's ditch the fad diets and discover the power of eating real, delicious food. Get ready to embrace a flavorful transformation, one grain at a time.

(Almost) Everyone Benefits:
Why This Plan Works.

Let's bust the myth that the Exotic Rice Hack is only suitable for a select few. The beauty of this approach lies in its inclusivity. Whether you're a college student juggling a packed schedule, a passionate home cook seeking culinary adventures, or someone navigating health challenges, rice holds the potential to be that delicious and nutritious foundation for a healthy lifestyle.

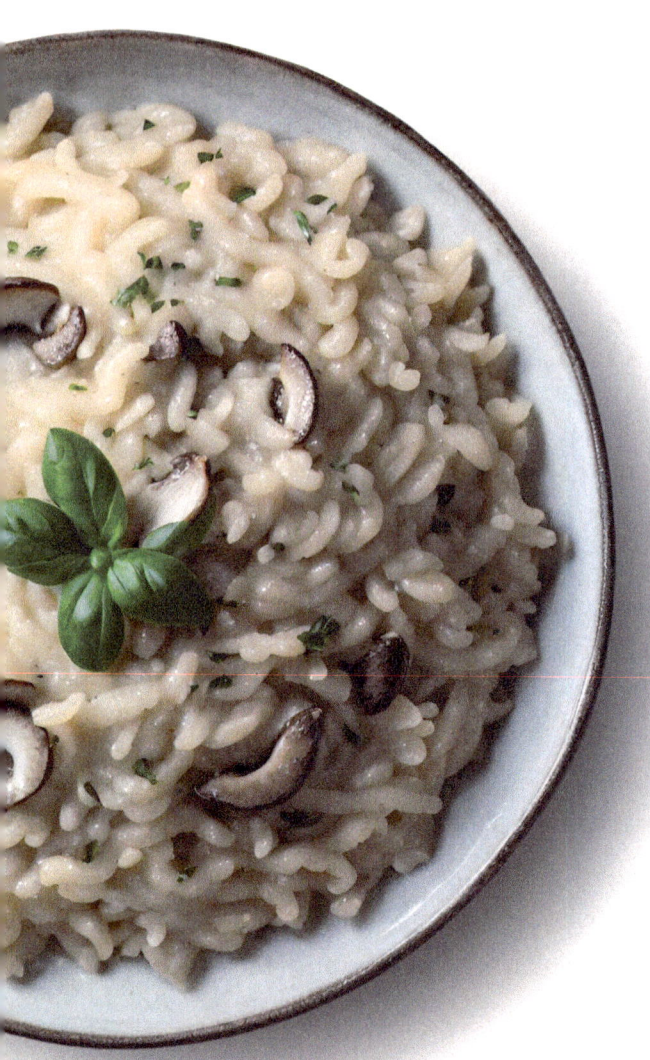

Picture this: You're a vegetarian always searching for new and satisfying plant-based meals. Turning to black beans with smoky chipotle-spiced brown rice for a vibrant protein punch becomes your go-to. Or perhaps, you crave rich flavors and comforting textures – Italian Arborio rice transforms into a creamy mushroom risotto that satisfies without leaving you feeling overly full or tired. And for the adventurers, that fragrant coconut milk-infused Thai Jasmine rice paired with a fiery mango salsa transports your taste buds straight to the tropics! The diverse world of rice has something for everyone, making it easier to stick to a plan that nourishes both your body and soul.

By embracing the philosophy of the Exotic Rice Hack, you're not only setting yourself up for success, but you're also minimizing the risk of falling into that dreaded "diet burnout." Unlike restrictive plans that leave you constantly craving "forbidden" foods, the abundance of flavor combinations and exciting cuisines within the rice world keep your meals engaging and delicious. This significantly reduces those urges to cheat or give up altogether, ultimately leading to more sustainable results.

If you're someone concerned about maintaining steady blood sugar levels, whether you have pre-diabetes or Type 2 diabetes, rice can be a smart strategic choice. Unlike refined carbohydrates found in sugary drinks, white bread, or processed snacks that cause dramatic blood sugar spikes and crashes, whole grains like brown rice, wild rice, and black rice deliver a treasure trove of fiber. This fiber slows the digestion of carbohydrates, allowing glucose to be released gradually into your bloodstream. This can contribute to improved blood sugar control, reducing the risk of energy crashes and constant hunger that can often sabotage wellness efforts.

Remember, managing blood sugar is complex, and portion sizes do matter! The magic lies in creating balanced meals that always feature a combination of complex carbohydrates (your delicious rice!), lean proteins, healthy fats (think avocado or a drizzle of olive oil), and plenty of vibrant, fiber-filled vegetables.

The essence of the Exotic Rice Hack is about shifting your mindset. It's about ditching the calorie-obsessed deprivation mentality and embracing the abundance and joy that delicious, nourishing foods can provide. With rice as your guide, you'll discover that eating for wellness can be both satisfying and sustainable – a recipe for true success!

Gluten-Free Goodness:
Your Natural Choice.

Rice shines even brighter for those seeking gluten-free options. Gluten, a protein found primarily in wheat, rye, and barley, can be problematic for a significant number of people. For those with Celiac disease, an autoimmune condition affecting roughly 1% of the population, even trace amounts of gluten can trigger a severe reaction. However, many individuals experience milder sensitivities to gluten that manifest as digestive discomfort, bloating, fatigue, and a whole host of vague, yet disruptive symptoms.

The beauty of rice lies in its natural gluten-free status. It offers a whole-food solution, making it a safe and delicious choice for those navigating a gluten-free diet. For many who find rice easy to digest, switching to rice-based meals can bring noticeable improvements in energy levels, digestion, and overall well-being. While gluten sensitivities can be challenging to diagnose, if you notice a positive shift after incorporating more rice and minimizing gluten-containing grains, it might be a sign that this change benefits your body.

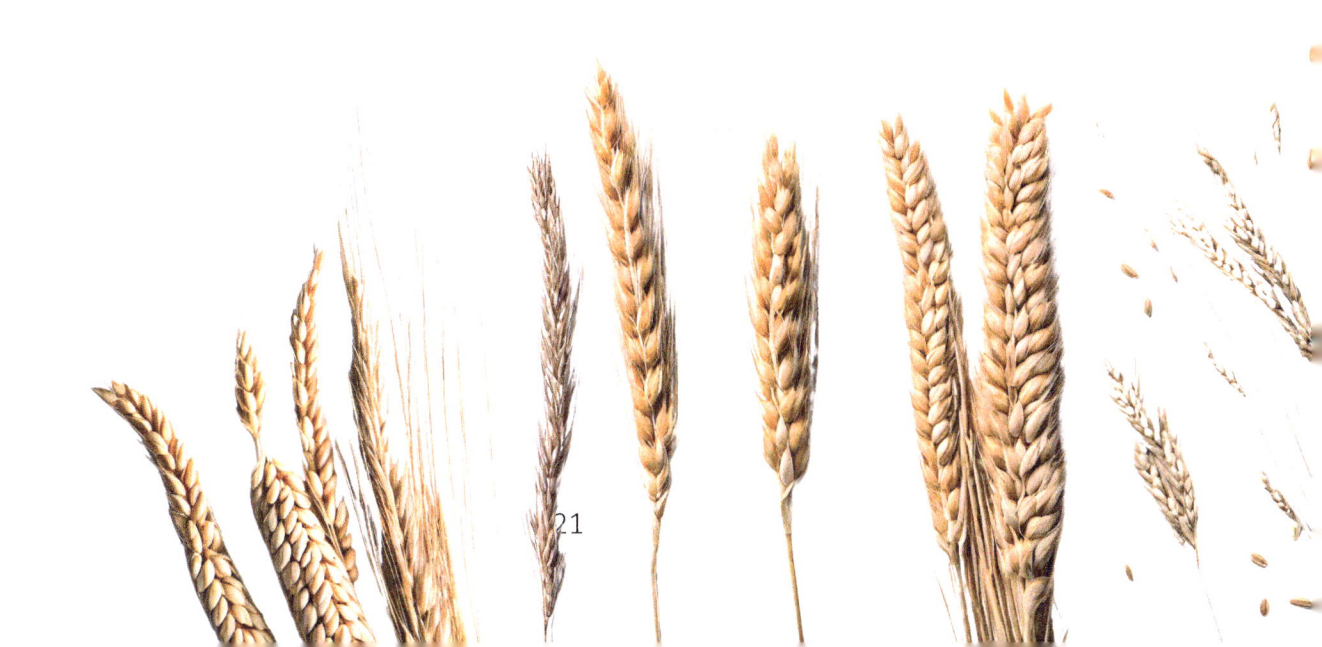

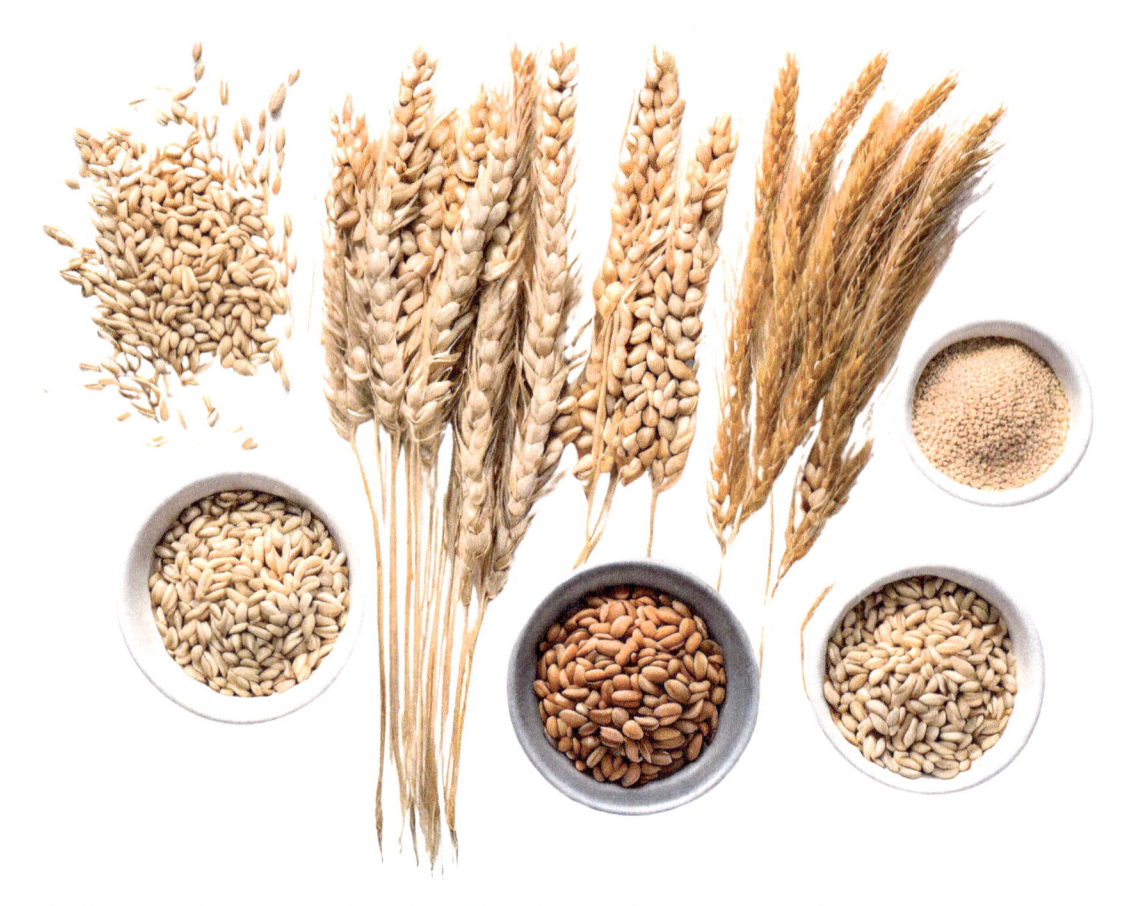

However, let's not make the mistake of thinking that all gluten-free products are created equal. Unfortunately, the rise in popularity of gluten-free diets has led to a flood of highly processed, gluten-free snacks and products. Often, these items are stripped of natural fiber and loaded with refined starches, sugars, and additives to mimic the taste and texture of gluten-containing foods. While convenient, they don't offer the same nutritional benefits as focusing on whole, unprocessed foods like rice.

This is where focusing on whole grain varieties of rice like brown, red, black, and wild rice really pays off. Not only are they naturally gluten-free, but also deliver a treasure trove of essential nutrients. Brown rice provides a good source of magnesium, crucial for energy production, and manganese, an important component of antioxidant systems that protect your cells. Red and black rice varieties contain anthocyanins, potent antioxidants linked to potential heart health and cognitive benefits. Swapping out a handful of gluten-free crackers for a satisfying bowl of red rice mixed with black beans and roasted vegetables is a win-win for both your tastebuds and overall health.

So, even if you don't have a diagnosed gluten intolerance or Celiac disease, the Exotic Rice Hack is a smart move towards a more nourishing diet. It encourages you to step away from processed foods, prioritize whole grains, and embrace the culinary creativity that rice inspires. You might be surprised at how much better you feel!

Adaptable Feasting:
Your Diet, Your Way.

Let's get ready to personalize your Exotic Rice Hack experience, unlocking a way of eating that's as delicious as it is sustainable! Embracing your individual preferences is key. Some thrive on the nutty flavor and slight chewiness of Himalayan Red Rice, while others might swoon over the intoxicating fragrance of Indian Basmati. There's room for everyone on this journey! Exploring the world of rice will undoubtedly lead you to your personal favorites, ensuring every meal is filled with flavors you genuinely crave.

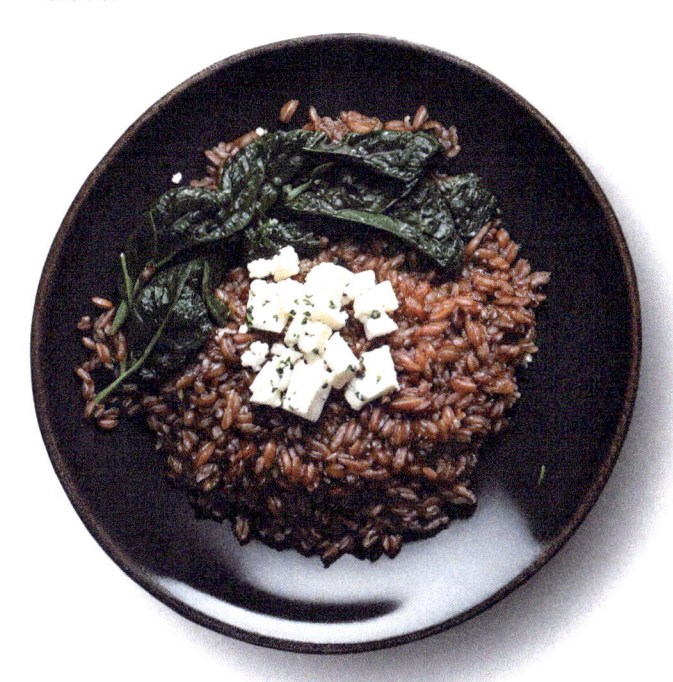

Now imagine opening your spice cabinet and refrigerator as gateways to culinary exploration. Think of rice as your blank canvas, awaiting a vibrant splash of flavors and textures. Start with a perfectly cooked pot of earthy Bhutanese Red Rice. A generous handful of garlicky sauteed spinach, a sprinkle of salty Greek feta cheese, and a drizzle of rich, lemon-infused olive oil take your taste buds straight to the Mediterranean with minimal effort. Or, transform leftover Arborio rice into a lusciously creamy rice pudding, adding a touch of warming vanilla extract, a sprinkle of Ceylon cinnamon, and a handful of sweet-tart dried cranberries.

Do not forget the power of leftovers in combating both food waste and the "I'm bored with this diet" blues. That extra cup of cooked brown rice finds new life as a "clean out your fridge" style fried rice. With a drizzle of toasted sesame oil, a splash of tamari (or soy sauce), a handful of chopped scallions, and a scramble of eggs, you have a flavorful, satisfying lunch in minutes. Or perhaps, chilled white rice becomes the foundation for a Mediterranean-inspired salad, with pops of color and flavor from juicy cherry tomatoes, Kalamata olives, crumbled feta, a sprinkle of dried oregano, and a zesty red wine vinaigrette.

The Exotic Rice Hack invites you to become a culinary adventurer and recipe remixer! Feel empowered to add your signature touches to dishes. Swap the brown rice in your favorite recipe for a vibrant mix of wild and red rice for a boost of visual appeal and texture. Or, if you're craving a creamy mushroom risotto but don't have any Arborio rice on hand, experiment with pearled barley for a satisfying, unexpected twist. Think back to how you viewed your diet prior to embarking on the Exotic Rice Hack. Perhaps the word "diet" itself conjured up feelings of deprivation and inevitable failure. But this way of eating is refreshingly different. It's about embracing flavor, flexibility, and the sheer joy of nourishing your body with real, vibrant food.

Rice becomes your trusted ally, a stepping stone to unlocking your culinary potential and a gateway to exciting new taste experiences. Whether you're drawn to the fluffy texture and subtle floral notes of Jasmine rice, the earthy nuttiness of wild rice, or the creamy comfort of Arborio, rice opens up a universe of possibilities. By choosing the varieties you truly enjoy, you transform a mundane meal into an experience to look forward to.

The best part? This plan is yours to shape. It honors your preferences and gives you the freedom to customize to your heart's content. Love spice? Let those curries simmer with fiery chilies, fragrant ginger, and the fresh vibrancy of herbs. Crave comfort? A classic risotto oozing with cheesy goodness and sprinkled with toasted pine nuts delivers warmth and satisfaction. And who said rice pudding is just for dessert? Garnished with toasted almonds, a drizzle of honey, and a dusting of cinnamon, it's a nourishing way to start your day.

Forget about obsessively counting calories or meticulously measuring portions. The Exotic Rice Hack encourages intuitive eating grounded in the hunger and fullness signals your body naturally provides. Prioritizing fiber-rich whole grains, colorful vegetables, and lean proteins creates a sense of satiety that prevents constant cravings and the urge to mindlessly overeat.

Adopting this new mindset allows you to say goodbye to the dreaded "diet burnout" cycle once and for all. You'll be too busy discovering delicious flavor combinations and experimenting with new recipes to feel deprived. The abundance of choices and the endless inspiration for transformation keeps boredom at bay, paving the way for a way of eating that feels both exciting and effortlessly sustainable.

The Exotic Rice Hack isn't just about transforming what's on your plate. It's about embracing nourishment as a source of joy, not punishment. It's about trusting your inner chef and discovering that healthy eating doesn't have to mean sacrifice. With each delicious bite, you'll be fueling your body, fueling your spirit, and creating a relationship with food that empowers you for life.

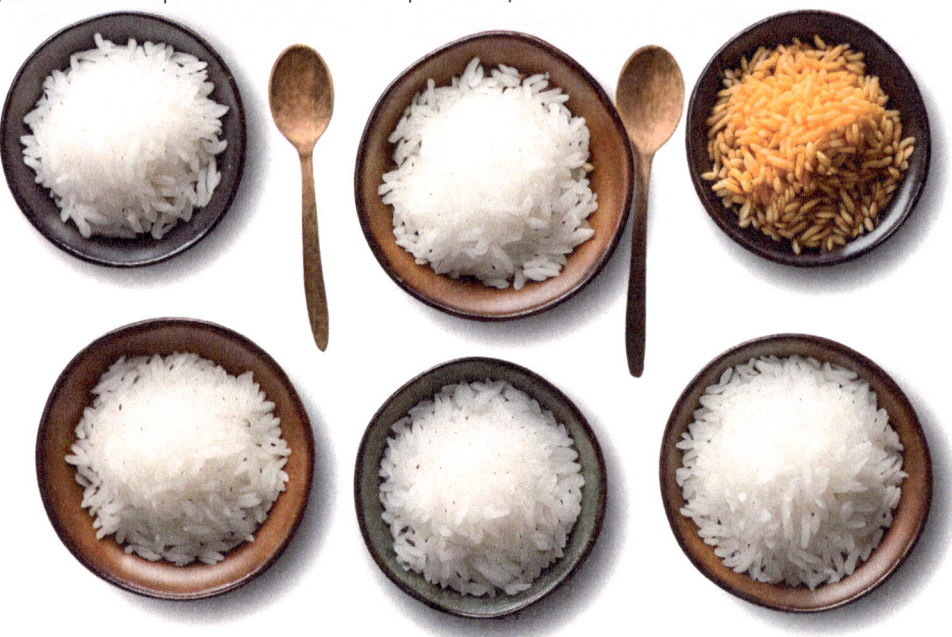

Rise and Shine
BREAKFAST

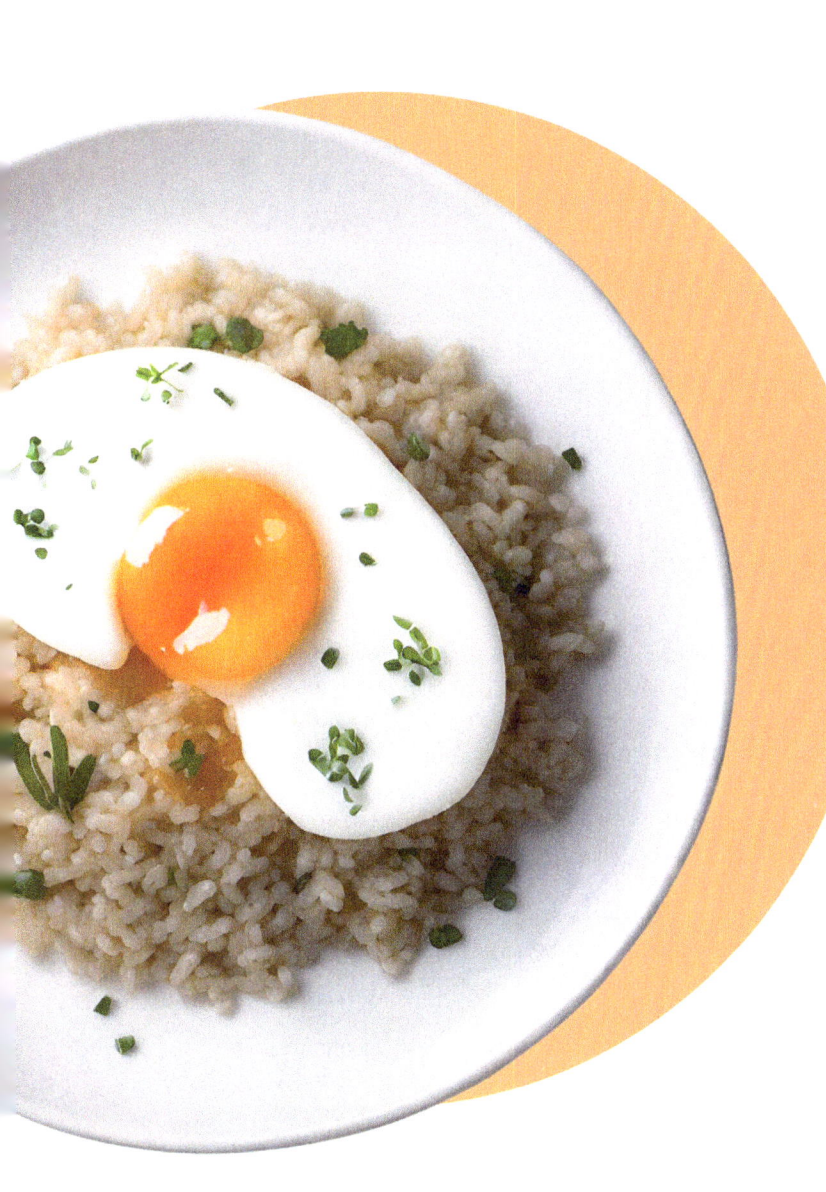

Mornings often feel rushed, leaving little room for culinary creativity. But what if breakfast could be a delicious adventure, a way to fuel your body and excite your tastebuds from the moment you wake up? Say goodbye to sad bowls of soggy cereal or flavorless oatmeal. It's time to transform your mornings with the power of rice!

This incredible grain isn't just for lunchtime or dinner; it's remarkably versatile and ready to elevate your breakfast game. Think creamy coconut rice porridge with exotic mango, savory rice omelets packed with vibrant veggies, or warm, comforting rice pudding with a swirl of cinnamon and honey. Rice can be a satisfying base for a global culinary journey right in your own kitchen.

Even with busy schedules, a delicious and nourishing breakfast is absolutely achievable. Discover the ease of make-ahead options like overnight rice puddings or flavorful breakfast fried rice that repurposes leftovers. Embrace rice's potential, and mornings will never be boring again. Get ready for breakfast to become your favorite meal of the day!

TROPICAL COCONUT RICE PORRIDGE

SERVES: 2 • PREP TIME: 5 MIN • COOK TIME: 15 MIN

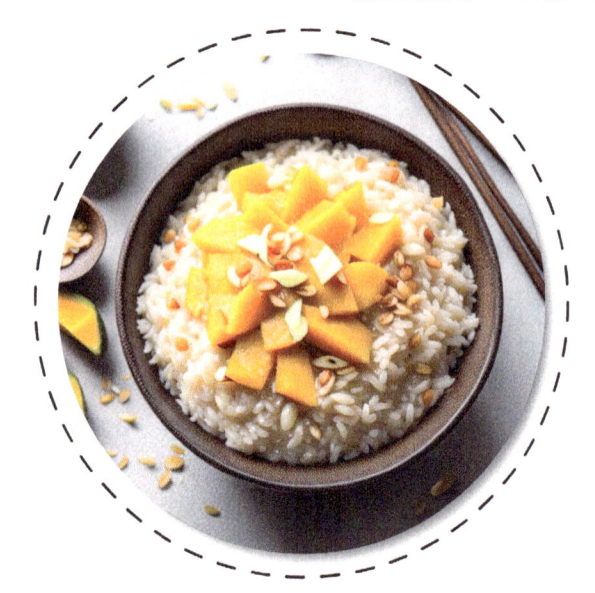

This porridge is packed with fiber, healthy fats, and natural sweetness for sustained energy. Brown rice delivers slow-release carbs, coconut milk adds fullness-boosting healthy fats, and mango provides sweetness and vitamins. This balanced breakfast helps prevent blood sugar crashes that can hinder weight loss.

NUTRITIONAL FACTS *(per serving)*

Calories: 260 **Protein**: 5 g
Carbohydrates: 40 g **Fat**: 12 g
Fiber: 6 g **Sugar**: 10 g

INGREDIENTS

- 1/4 cup diced fresh mango (about half a mango)
- 2 tablespoons toasted coconut flakes
- 1 cup cooked brown rice (make ahead for quick prep)
- 1 cup unsweetened coconut milk
- 1/2 cup water
- 1/4 teaspoon ground cinnamon

INSTRUCTIONS

1. Select a ripe mango that yields slightly to gentle pressure. Carefully slice in half, avoiding the large central pit. Score the flesh into a grid pattern and scoop out the mango cubes with a spoon. Set aside.

2. (Optional) For maximum flavor, spread the coconut flakes in a thin layer in a dry skillet. Toast over medium-low heat, stirring constantly for 2-3 minutes, or until lightly browned and fragrant. Remove from heat and set aside.

3. In a medium saucepan, add the pre-cooked brown rice, unsweetened coconut milk, water, and ground cinnamon.

4. Place the saucepan over medium heat and bring the mixture to a gentle simmer. Stir frequently to prevent sticking and achieve a creamy consistency.

5. Cook the porridge for approximately 10-15 minutes. The exact time will depend on your desired consistency. If you prefer a thicker porridge, continue cooking for a few additional minutes.

6. Once the porridge has reached your desired thickness, remove it from the heat. Gently fold in the diced mango, taking care to not completely mush the fruit.

7. Divide the porridge into two bowls. Sprinkle each serving with the toasted coconut flakes for a delightful crunch.

MEDITERRANEAN SRAMBLE

SERVES: 2 • PREP TIME: 5 MIN • COOK TIME: 5-8 MIN

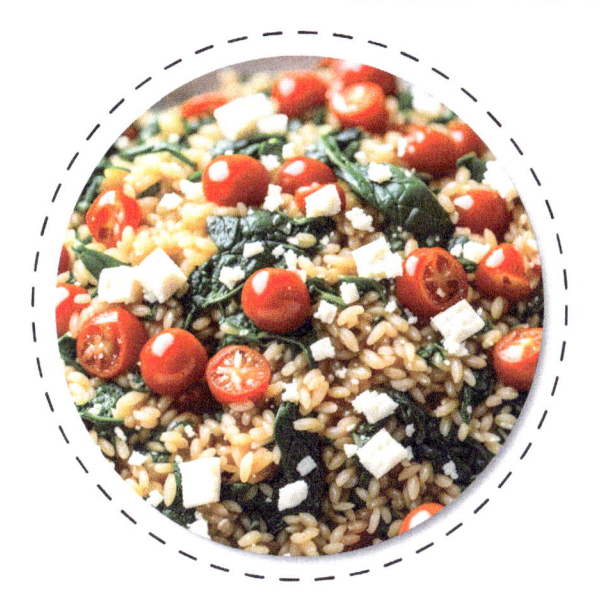

This scramble is packed with nutrients for weight loss! Leftover rice provides fiber for steady energy, while spinach offers vitamins and iron. Tomatoes add sweetness and antioxidants, feta delivers a salty boost, and Greek yogurt increases protein for lasting fullness.

NUTRITIONAL FACTS *(per serving)*

Calories: 250
Carbohydrates: 28g
Fiber: 4 g
Protein: 10 g
Fat: 14 g
Sugar: 5 g

INGREDIENTS

- 1 tablespoon olive oil
- 1 cup chopped fresh spinach
- 1/2 cup halved cherry tomatoes
- 1 cup cooked rice (any variety, leftover is perfect!)
- 1/4 cup crumbled feta cheese
- Salt and black pepper to taste
- Greek yogurt for serving (optional)

INSTRUCTIONS

1. Thoroughly wash and dry the spinach leaves. If using large leaves, roughly chop them for easier eating. Cut the cherry tomatoes in half lengthwise.

2. Place a medium skillet over medium heat and add the olive oil.

3. Once the oil shimmers, add the spinach to the pan. Cook for 1-2 minutes, stirring frequently until the spinach wilts and reduces in size.

4. Add the halved cherry tomatoes to the skillet along with the cooked rice. Stir to combine and heat everything through, about 2 minutes.

5. Season with a pinch of salt and black pepper to taste. Crumble the feta cheese over the scramble.

6. Divide the scramble onto plates. If desired, add a dollop of Greek yogurt to each serving for an extra

SAVORY RICE OMELET

SERVES: 2 • PREP TIME: 5 MIN • COOK TIME: 15 MIN

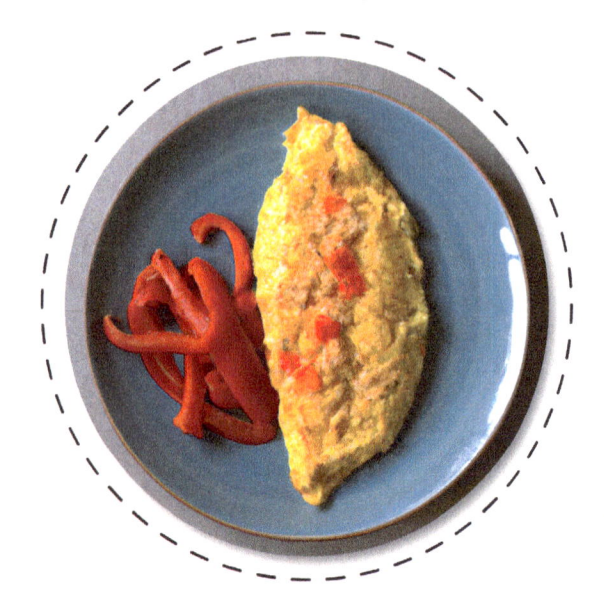

This omelet is packed with protein, fiber, and a satisfying variety of flavors, perfect for fueling your morning and preventing hunger pangs. Eggs provide high-quality protein, while brown rice adds complex carbohydrates and fiber to keep you feeling full. The addition of sauteed vegetables boosts vitamin content and adds an extra serving of fiber to your meal.

NUTRITIONAL FACTS *(per serving)*

Calories: 280 **Protein**: 18g
Carbohydrates: 25g **Fat**: 4 g
Fiber: 4 g **Sugar**: 3 g

INGREDIENTS

- 1 tablespoon olive oil
- 1 cup chopped fresh spinach
- 1/2 cup halved cherry tomatoes
- 1 cup cooked rice (any variety, leftover is perfect!)
- 1/4 cup crumbled feta cheese
- Salt and black pepper to taste
- Greek yogurt for serving (optional)

INSTRUCTIONS

1. Thoroughly wash and dry the bell peppers. Remove the seeds and stem, then chop into small pieces. Dice the onion.

2. Heat the olive oil in a medium skillet over medium heat. Add the chopped bell peppers and onion. Sauté for 3-5 minutes, stirring occasionally, until the vegetables soften.

3. Add the cooked brown rice to the pan with the sauteed vegetables. Stir to combine and allow the rice to warm through for 1-2 minutes.

4. In a separate bowl, whisk together the eggs, a tablespoon of water or milk (for fluffier eggs, optional), paprika, salt, and black pepper.

5. Lightly grease a nonstick skillet over medium-low heat. Pour the egg mixture into the preheated skillet. As the edges begin to set, gently lift them with a spatula, tilting the pan to allow the uncooked egg to flow underneath.

6. When the omelet is mostly set but still slightly runny on top, carefully add the rice and vegetable mixture to one half. Gently fold the other half of the omelet over the filling.

7. Cook for an additional 1-2 minutes until the egg is completely set and cooked through. Slide the omelet onto a plate and enjoy immediately!

BERRYLICIOUS RICE PUDDING PARFAIT

SERVES: 2 • PREP TIME: 10 MIN (+CHILLING TIME)

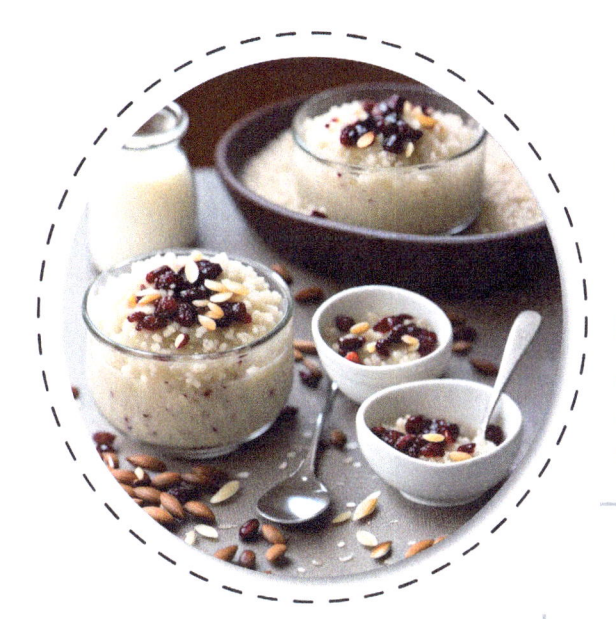

This parfait offers a balanced combination of complex carbohydrates from brown rice, healthy fats from almonds, and natural sweetness from dried cranberries. The fiber in the rice and cranberries helps you feel satisfied, while the protein in the almonds adds staying power to prevent blood sugar spikes and crashes.

NUTRITIONAL FACTS *(per serving)*

Calories: 320 **Protein**: 8 g
Carbohydrates: 50 g **Fat**: 15 g
Fiber: 7 g **Sugar**: 15 g

INGREDIENTS

- 1 cup cooked brown rice (chilled)
- 1 cup unsweetened vanilla almond milk
- 1/4 cup dried cranberries
- 1/4 cup chopped almonds
- 1/4 teaspoon vanilla extract
- Pinch of cinnamon

INSTRUCTIONS

1. Use individual glass jars, small bowls, or any resealable container for your parfaits.
2. Divide half of the cooked rice between your chosen containers. Next, add half of the vanilla almond milk, dividing it between the containers.
3. Sprinkle half of the dried cranberries and half the chopped almonds on top of the almond milk layer.
4. Repeat the layering process, adding the remaining rice, almond milk, cranberries, and almonds.
5. (Optional) If you desire, add a touch of vanilla extract and a sprinkle of cinnamon to each container.
6. Cover or seal your parfaits and place them in the refrigerator to chill overnight (or for at least a few hours). The next morning, you have a delicious, grab-and-go breakfast ready and waiting!

SOUTHWEST SUNRISE BOWL

SERVES: 2 • PREP TIME: 5 MIN (+VEGGIE PREP)

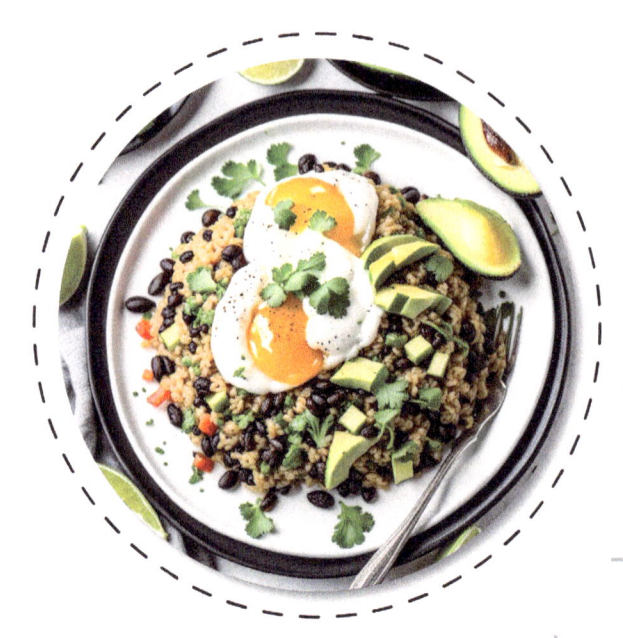

This bowl is packed with nutrients that support weight loss goals. Black beans and brown rice provide a satisfying combination of fiber and complex carbohydrates for steady energy release. Sliced avocado offers healthy fats to boost satiety, while salsa adds a pop of flavor with minimal calories. The poached egg delivers a rich dose of protein, keeping you feeling full and preventing cravings.

NUTRITIONAL FACTS *(per serving)*

Calories: 450   **Protein**: 22 g
Carbohydrates: 55 g   **Fat**: 20 g
Fiber: 15 g   **Sugar**: 5 g

INGREDIENTS

- 1 poached egg
- 1 cup cooked brown rice (warm or chilled)
- 1/2 cup cooked or canned black beans
- 1/2 cup salsa (your favorite variety)
- 1/4 avocado, sliced
- Hot sauce (optional)
- Fresh cilantro for garnish (optional)

INSTRUCTIONS

1. Poach your egg: There are numerous methods for perfectly poached eggs (search online for tutorials). A simple method is to bring a pot of water with a splash of vinegar to a gentle simmer, crack your egg into a small bowl, then gently slide it into the water and cook for 3-4 minutes until the white is set but the yolk remains runny.

2. Start with a base of warm or chilled brown rice. Top with a generous scoop of black beans and your favorite salsa.

3. Fan out the sliced avocado on top of your bowl.

4. Carefully place your poached egg in the center of the bowl.

5. Customize it! Add a drizzle of hot sauce if you like extra spice, and garnish with fresh cilantro for a vibrant touch.

PROTEIN-PACKED FRIED RICE

SERVES: 2   •   PREP TIME: 5 MIN   •   COOK TIME: 15 MIN

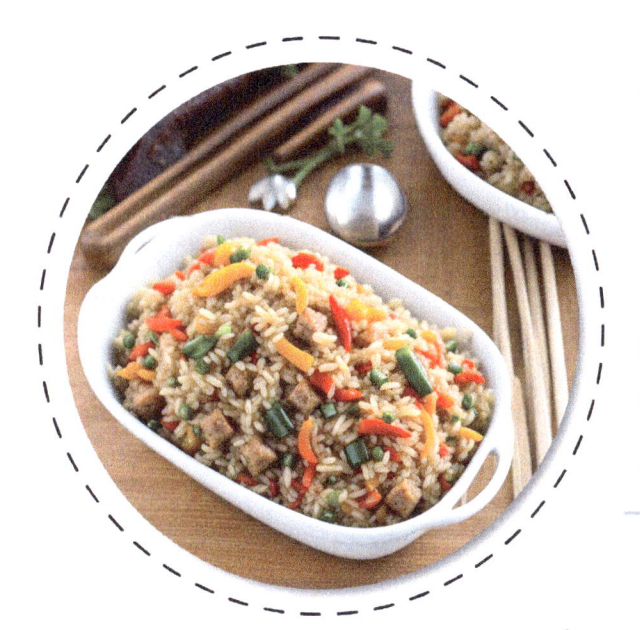

This fried rice delivers a winning combination of lean protein, complex carbohydrates, and a boost of veggies — ideal for fueling your morning. The protein from the sausage will keep you feeling full, the rice provides sustained energy, and the vegetables add vitamins, minerals, and extra fiber to the mix.

NUTRITIONAL FACTS *(per serving)*

Calories: 400
Carbohydrates: 35 g
Fiber: 4 g
Protein: 30 g
Fat: 20 g
Sugar: 4 g

INGREDIENTS

- 1 tablespoon olive oil (or preferred cooking oil)
- 1/2 cup diced lean turkey breakfast sausage
- 1/2 cup chopped vegetables (ex: onion, bell peppers, mushrooms)
- 2 cups cooked rice (any variety, leftover is great!)
- 2 large eggs, lightly beaten
- 1-2 tablespoons soy sauce, to taste
- Green onions for garnish (optional)

INSTRUCTIONS

1. Dice your onions, peppers, or other vegetables of choice. Slice the green onions (if using) for garnish.

2. Heat the olive oil in a large skillet or wok over medium-high heat. Add the diced sausage and cook until browned, breaking it up into small pieces. Add vegetables and cook for an additional 2-3 minutes, or until softened.

3. Add the cooked rice to the skillet and stir to combine with the sausage and vegetables. Create a well in the center of the pan and pour in the beaten eggs. Scramble the eggs until cooked, then toss to combine with the rice mixture.

4. Drizzle soy sauce over the fried rice, adding to taste. Garnish with sliced green onions (optional) and enjoy immediately.

APPLE-CINNAMON RICE BAKE

SERVES: 2   •   PREP TIME: 10 MIN   •   COOK TIME: 25 MIN

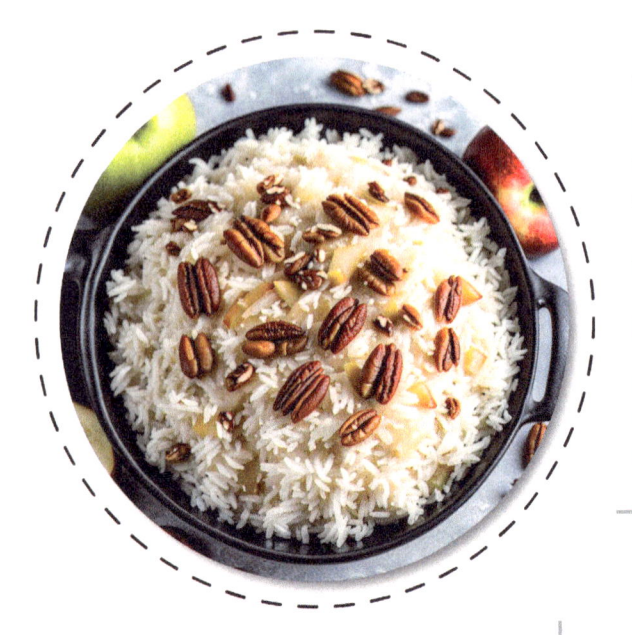

This baked breakfast offers balanced nutrition. The basmati rice and grated apple provide fiber and complex carbohydrates, while the hint of maple syrup adds natural sweetness. Pecans contribute healthy fats and a touch of protein, enhancing satiety. The warming cinnamon adds flavor without additional calories.

NUTRITIONAL FACTS *(per serving)*

Calories: 350   **Protein**: 6 g
Carbohydrates: 35 g   **Fat**: 15 g
Fiber: 6 g   **Sugar**: 20 g

INGREDIENTS

- 1 cup cooked basmati rice (warm or chilled)
- 1 medium apple, peeled and grated
- 2 tablespoons maple syrup
- 1 teaspoon ground cinnamon
- 1/4 cup chopped pecans
- Pinch of salt
- 2 tablespoons milk or plant-based milk (optional)

INSTRUCTIONS

1. Preheat your oven: Set your oven to 375°F (190°C) and lightly grease a small baking dish.

2. Combine ingredients: In a medium bowl, mix the cooked basmati rice, grated apple, maple syrup, cinnamon, chopped pecans, and a pinch of salt.

3. Optional: For a richer, creamier bake, add 2 tablespoons of milk (or your preferred plant-based alternative) to the mixture.

4. Pour the rice mixture into the prepared baking dish. Bake for 20-25 minutes, or until the top is golden brown and the bake is bubbly. Serve warm.

PEANUT BUTTER BOWL

SERVES: 2 • PREP TIME: 5 MIN • COOK TIME: 0 MIN

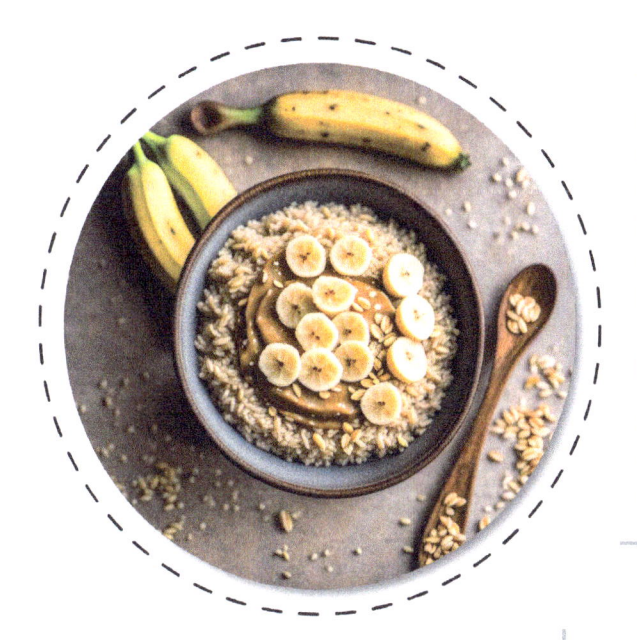

This bowl packs a balanced punch of complex carbohydrates, protein, healthy fats, and fiber. Brown rice delivers sustained energy, while peanut butter and hemp seeds provide protein and satisfying fats to keep you feeling full. The banana adds natural sweetness and extra nutrients, while the drizzle of honey offers a touch of indulgence while keeping overall sugar content in check.

NUTRITIONAL FACTS *(per serving)*

Calories: 450　　**Protein**: 12 g
Carbohydrates: 65 g　　**Fat**: 22 g
Fiber: 8 g　　**Sugar**: 25 g

INGREDIENTS

- 1 cup cooked brown rice (warm)
- 1 tablespoon peanut butter (smooth or crunchy)
- 1/2 banana, sliced
- 1 teaspoon honey
- 1 tablespoon hemp seeds

INSTRUCTIONS

1. Warm the rice: If your cooked brown rice has been refrigerated, warm it gently in a saucepan or the microwave.

2. Assemble your bowl: Place the warm rice in a bowl. Swirl a spoonful of peanut butter into the rice. Top with banana slices and drizzle with honey.

3. Add the final touch: Sprinkle hemp seeds over the bowl for an extra boost of healthy fats and a satisfying crunch. Enjoy immediately!

HUMMUS & VEGGIE RICE WRAPS

SERVES: 4 WRAPS • PREP TIME: 10 MIN • COOK TIME: 25 MIN

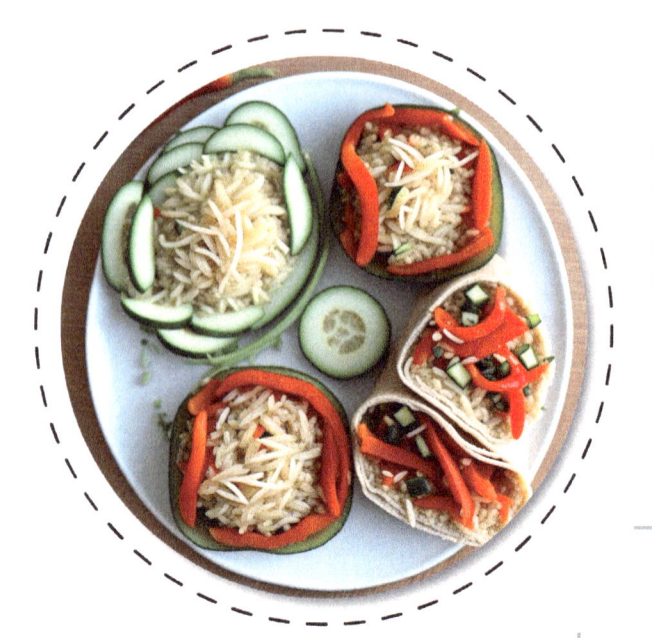

This wrap is packed with fiber, protein, and healthy fats, making it both delicious and supportive of your weight loss goals. Hummus offers protein and satisfying fats from chickpeas, while whole wheat tortillas and brown rice deliver complex carbs and fiber for steady energy. The roasted red peppers, cucumbers, and sprouts add an abundance of vitamins, minerals, and additional fiber.

NUTRITIONAL FACTS *(per serving)*

Calories: 300
Carbohydrates: 45 g
Fiber: 8 g
Protein: 10 g
Fat: 12 g
Sugar: 5 g

INGREDIENTS

- 1/2 cup roasted red peppers, sliced
- 1/2 cucumber, sliced
- 4 whole-wheat tortillas (medium size)
- 1/2 cup prepared hummus
- 1 cup cooked brown rice (chilled)
- 1/2 cup sprouts (alfalfa, radish, etc.)

INSTRUCTIONS

1. Prep the veggies: Slice your cucumber into thin rounds. If your roasted red peppers are whole, slice them into strips.

2. Assemble the wraps: Lay out each tortilla. Spread a thin layer of hummus evenly over the surface. Top with a scoop of cooked brown rice, leaving a border around the edge. Arrange a layer of roasted red peppers, cucumber slices, and a handful of sprouts.

3. Roll and enjoy: Tightly roll up each tortilla, tucking in the sides as you roll. Cut the wraps in half for easy eating, or leave them whole. Enjoy immediately or wrap them in parchment paper or foil for a packed lunch.

SWEET POTATO RICE PUDDING CUPS

SERVES: 2 • PREP TIME: 10 MIN • COOK TIME: 0 MIN

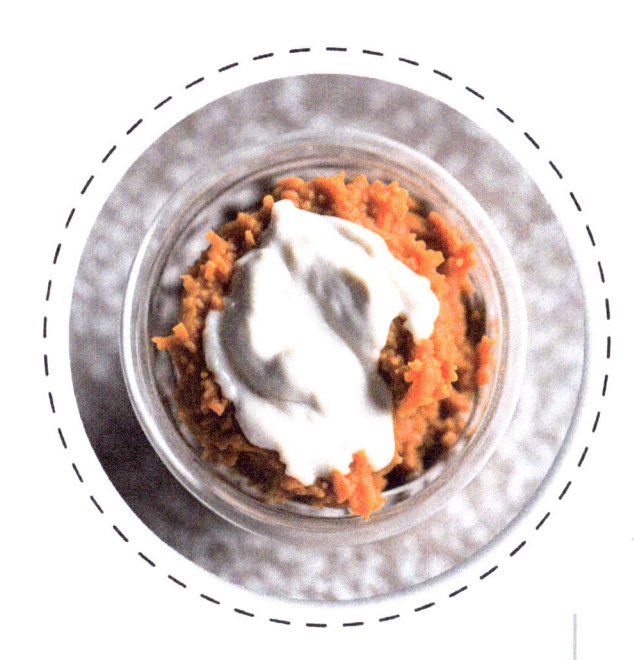

This dessert satisfies sweet cravings without sabotaging your weight loss goals. Sweet potato offers a generous dose of vitamin A and fiber, while the Greek yogurt contributes protein for satiety. The pre-cooked rice adds bulk, and the sliced almonds offer healthy fats and a touch of crunch. This delicious treat allows for a hint of indulgence while staying on track.

NUTRITIONAL FACTS *(per serving)*

Calories: 450
Carbohydrates: 65 g
Fiber: 8 g
Protein: 12 g
Fat: 22 g
Sugar: 25 g

INGREDIENTS

- 1 cup cooked sweet potato, mashed
- 1 cup cooked rice (any variety)
- 1/2 cup plain Greek yogurt
- 1 teaspoon vanilla extract
- 1/4 teaspoon ground nutmeg
- 2 tablespoons sliced almonds

INSTRUCTIONS

1. Mash the sweet potato: Make sure the sweet potato is cooked until tender and easily mashed.

2. Build your layers: Divide the mashed sweet potato between small glass jars, bowls, or ramekins. Top with a layer of pre-cooked rice, then add a dollop of Greek yogurt to each cup.

3. Flavor and Finish: Sprinkle a dash of nutmeg and a pinch of vanilla extract (optional) over each cup. To finish, add a sprinkle of sliced almonds to each serving.

4. Chill and enjoy: For the best flavor and texture, cover and refrigerate the cups for at least an hour (or overnight).

BANANA-NUT RICE PANCAKES

SERVES: 4-5 PANCAKES • PREP TIME: 10 MIN • COOK TIME: 10 MIN

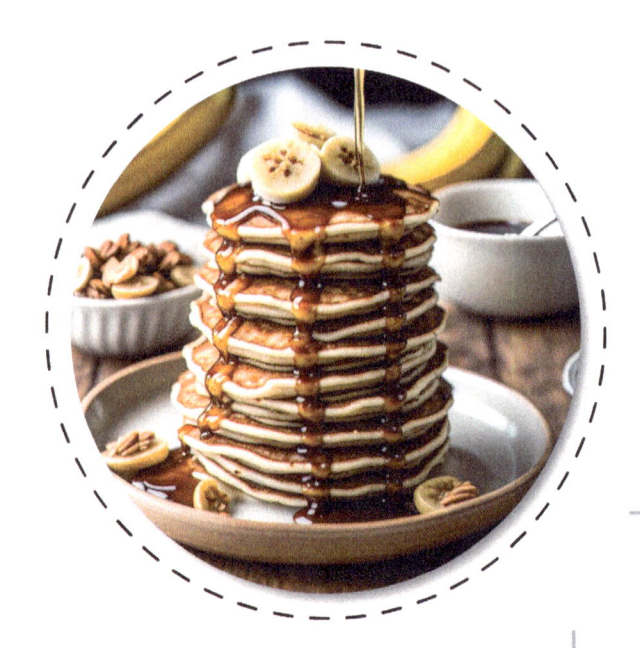

These pancakes are a champion for weight management goals. Brown rice flour offers a source of complex carbohydrates for sustained energy, while mashed banana provides natural sweetness and keeps you feeling full. The addition of eggs contributes protein, and chopped walnuts add healthy fats to further enhance satiety and prevent blood sugar spikes.

NUTRITIONAL FACTS *(per serving)*

Calories: 180
Carbohydrates: 25 g
Fiber: 2 g
Protein: 5 g
Fat: 8 g
Sugar: 5 g

INGREDIENTS

- 1 cup brown rice flour
- 1/2 teaspoon ground cinnamon (optional)
- Pinch of salt
- 1 ripe banana, mashed
- 1 teaspoon vanilla extract
- 2 large eggs
- 1/4 cup chopped walnuts
- Coconut oil or cooking oil for greasing the pan

INSTRUCTIONS

1. In a medium bowl, whisk together the brown rice flour, cinnamon (if using), and salt.

2. In a separate bowl, mash the ripe banana. Add the eggs and vanilla extract to the mashed banana and whisk until well combined.

3. Pour the wet ingredients into the dry ingredients and stir until just combined. Be careful not to overmix, a few lumps are okay!

4. Gently fold in the chopped walnuts, ensuring they are evenly distributed throughout the batter.

5. Heat a lightly oiled griddle or frying pan over medium heat. Once hot, pour about 1/4 cup of batter for each pancake.

6. Cook the pancakes for 2-3 minutes per side, or until golden brown and cooked through. You can peek underneath to check for doneness – if the edges look set, it's probably time to flip!

7. Serve your Banana-Nut Rice Pancakes immediately while they're warm and fluffy. Enjoy them on their own, or drizzle with a touch of maple syrup or your favorite topping.

FRUITY RICE SALAD

SERVES: 2 • PREP TIME: 10 MIN • COOK TIME: 0 MIN

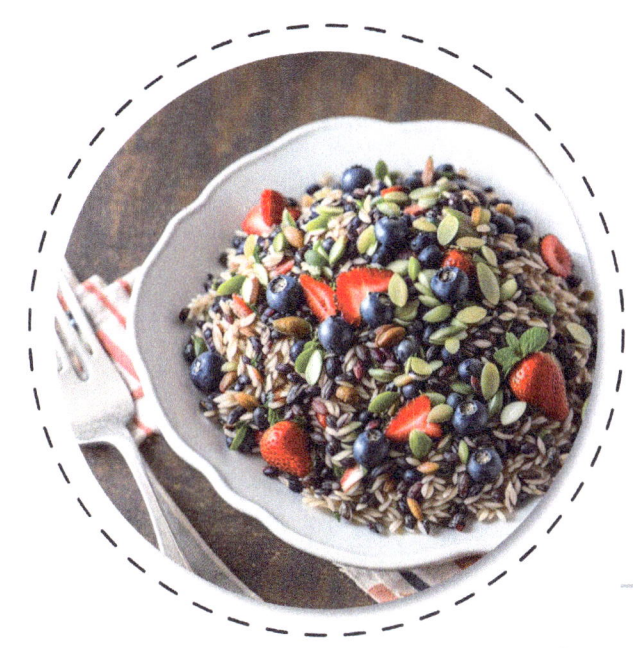

This salad is a nutritional powerhouse that'll keep you full while supporting your weight loss goals. Wild rice provides complex carbohydrates and fiber for steady energy and satiety, while blueberries and strawberries are packed with antioxidants and natural sweetness. Toasted pumpkin seeds offer a source of healthy fats and protein, and the honey-lemon vinaigrette adds a touch of tangy brightness without

NUTRITIONAL FACTS *(per serving)*

Calories: 180
Carbohydrates: 25 g
Fiber: 2 g
Protein: 5 g
Fat: 8 g
Sugar: 5 g

INGREDIENTS

- 1/2 cup fresh blueberries
- 1/2 cup chopped strawberries
- 2 tablespoons olive oil
- 1 tablespoon lemon juice
- 1 teaspoon honey
- Pinch of salt
- Pinch of black pepper
- 1/4 cup toasted pumpkin seeds
- 1 cup cooked wild rice (chilled)

INSTRUCTIONS

1. Thoroughly wash the blueberries and strawberries. Hull and chop the strawberries into bite-sized pieces.

2. Make the dressing: In a small bowl, whisk together the olive oil, lemon juice, honey, salt, and pepper until well combined.

3. In a medium bowl, combine the cooked wild rice, blueberries, strawberries, and toasted pumpkin seeds. Pour the dressing over the salad and gently toss to evenly coat.

4. Serve immediately for the best texture, or chill in the refrigerator for a refreshing later snack or meal.

TURMERIC GOLDEN MILK RICE PUDDING

SERVES: 2 • PREP TIME: 10 MIN • COOK TIME: 15 MIN

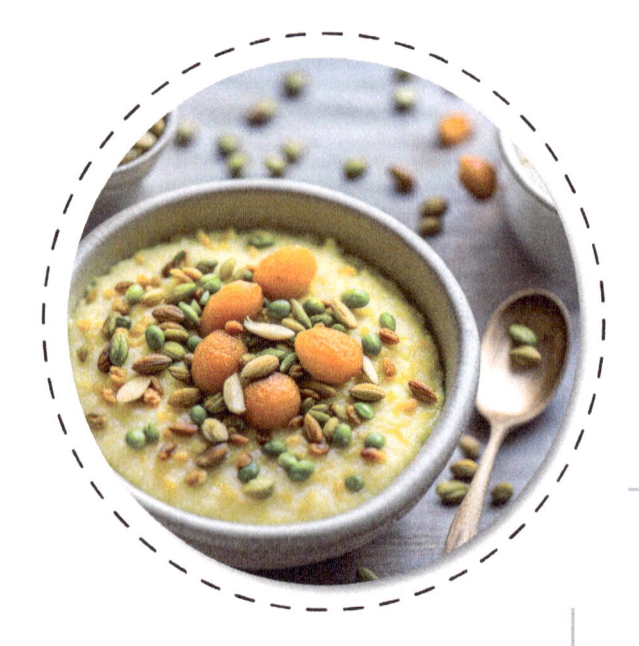

This rice pudding offers a delicious way to incorporate anti-inflammatory spices while still feeling like an indulgence. Basmati rice provides complex carbohydrates for energy, while coconut milk offers healthy fats for satiety. The natural sweetness from honey keeps the overall sugar content in check, and the vibrant spices like turmeric and ginger support healthy digestion.

NUTRITIONAL FACTS *(per serving)*

Calories: 380
Carbohydrates: 55 g
Fiber: 4 g
Protein: 6 g
Fat: 20 g
Sugar: 25 g

INGREDIENTS

- 1 cup cooked basmati rice (warm or chilled)
- 1 cup unsweetened coconut milk
- 1/2 cup water
- 1/2 teaspoon ground turmeric
- 1/4 teaspoon ground ginger
- 1 tablespoon honey
- 1/4 cup chopped pistachios
- 1/4 cup chopped dried apricots

INSTRUCTIONS

1. In a medium saucepan, combine the cooked basmati rice, coconut milk, water, turmeric, and ginger. Bring the mixture to a gentle simmer over medium-low heat.

2. Stir in the honey and continue to simmer for 10-15 minutes, or until the pudding thickens to your desired consistency. Stir occasionally to prevent sticking.

3. Remove the saucepan from the heat and let the pudding cool slightly before dividing it into serving bowls or cups.

4. Top each serving with a sprinkle of chopped pistachios and dried apricots. Enjoy warm or chill for a refreshing treat.

Lunchtime
LEGENDS

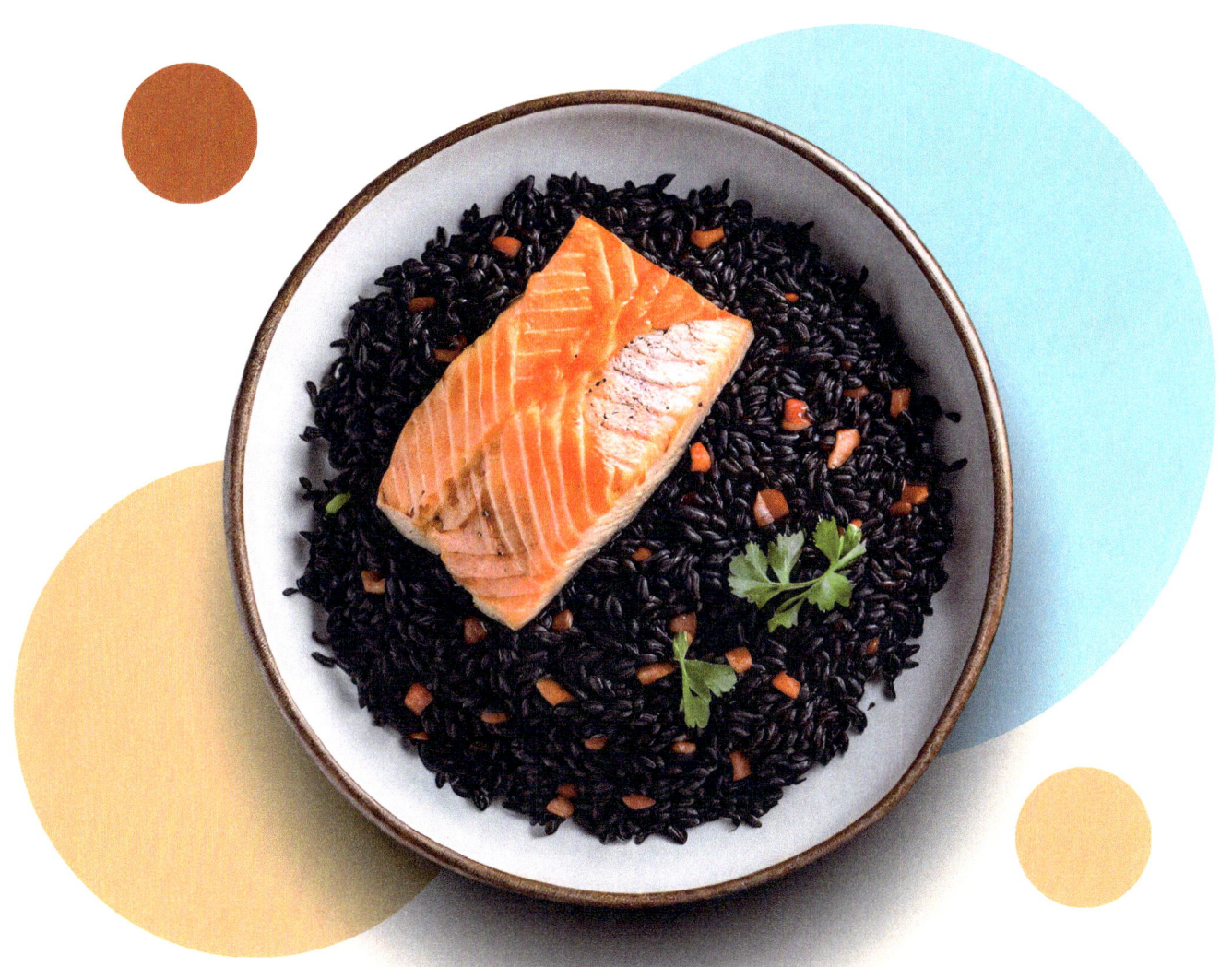

Forget boring lunches! It's time for a rice revolution. This globally-loved grain is so much more than a side dish – it's a nutritional star with tons of flavor potential. From fragrant basmati to nutty brown rice, each type offers something delicious. Think vibrant Mediterranean bowls, Thai curries, and so much more! Rice is budget-friendly, satisfying, and packed with goodness (hello fiber and antioxidants!). It's your blank canvas for flavor - herbs, spices, and global cuisines pair perfectly. Say goodbye to lunchtime blahs and hello to exciting, healthy meals. Get ready to discover why rice makes lunch legendary!

ASIAN STIR-FRY DELIGHT

SERVES: 2 • PREP TIME: 10 MIN • COOK TIME: 20 MIN

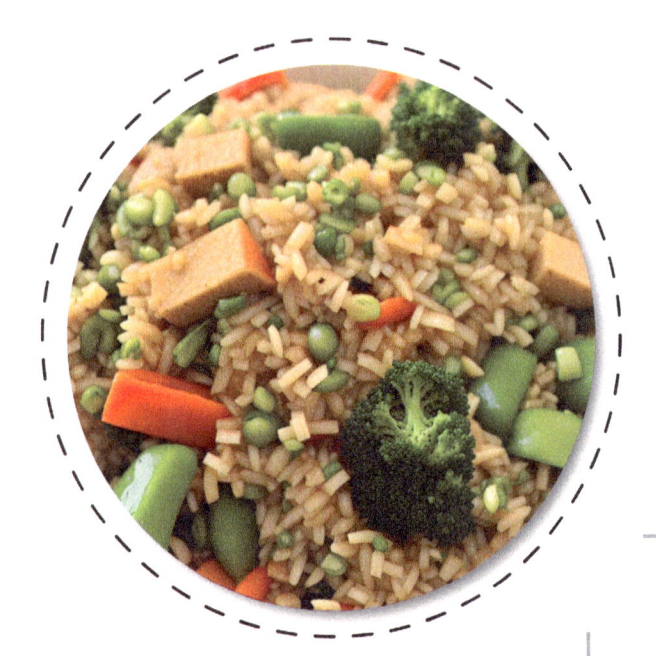

This recipe combines nutty brown rice, your favorite lean protein, and a vibrant mix of crisp vegetables, all tossed in a savory, light sauce made with soy sauce and sesame oil. Brown rice provides filling fiber, while your choice of chicken, tofu, or shrimp adds a boost of protein. The abundance of colorful vegetables delivers essential vitamins, minerals, and antioxidants. Plus, the flavorful sauce uses low-sodium soy sauce to keep the dish light and healthy.

NUTRITIONAL FACTS *(per serving)*

Calories: 350
Carbohydrates: 35 g
Fiber: 6 g
Protein: 25 g
Fat: 15 g
Sugar: 5 g

INGREDIENTS

- 1 cup cooked brown rice (1 to 1 1/2 cups uncooked)
- 1/2 pound protein (4 to 6 ounces chicken, tofu, or shrimp)
- 1 cup assorted vegetables (diced broccoli, bell peppers, carrots, snow peas)
- 1 tablespoon vegetable oil (or preferred cooking oil)
- 1 tablespoon low-sodium soy sauce
- 1 teaspoon sesame oil
- Optional: sesame seeds, green onions, red pepper flakes

INSTRUCTIONS

1. Cook the rice: Follow the instructions on the brown rice package. Typically this involves simmering 1 to 1 1/2 cups of uncooked rice in a medium saucepan with water for 20-30 minutes.

2. Cut the chicken (or prepare tofu or shrimp) into bite-sized pieces. Wash and chop assorted vegetables into similar-sized pieces.

3. Place the wok or skillet over medium-high heat. Add vegetable oil and let it heat up.

4. Add the protein to the hot pan. Cook for several minutes, stirring frequently until browned on all sides and cooked through. Remove from the pan.

5. Add the vegetables to the pan. Stir-fry for 2-3 minutes, or until crisp-tender.

6. Return the protein to the pan. Add the cooked brown rice. Drizzle with soy sauce and sesame oil. Gently toss to combine.

7. (Optional) Divide the stir-fry between bowls. Top with sesame seeds, green onions, or red pepper flakes if desired.

MEDITERRANEAN WILD RICE BOWL

SERVES: 2 • PREP TIME: 10 MIN • COOK TIME: 20 MIN

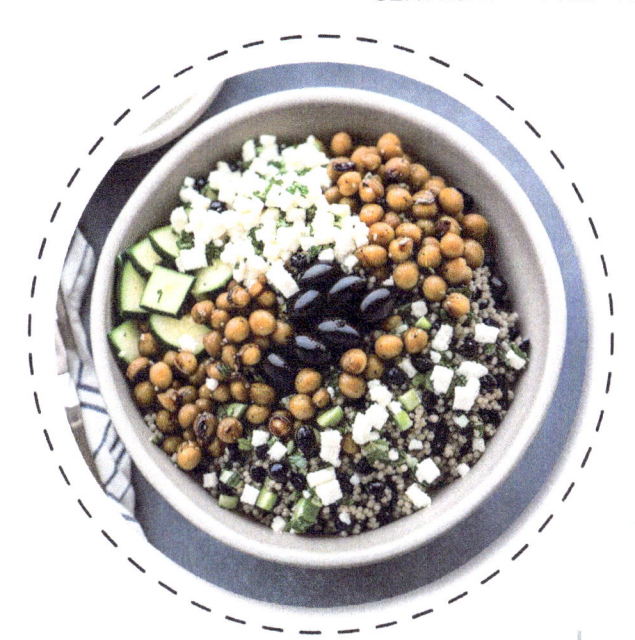

This Mediterranean Wild Rice Bowl is a vibrant and satisfying lunch option that delivers a perfect balance of flavor and nutrition. Wild rice provides a hearty dose of fiber, keeping you feeling full while roasted chickpeas add even more fiber and protein. Kalamata olives offer healthy fats, while the fresh cucumber and lemon vinaigrette contribute vitamins, antioxidants, and a burst of zesty flavor without excess calories.

NUTRITIONAL FACTS *(per serving)*

Calories: 380
Carbohydrates: 35 g
Fiber: 6 g
Protein: 8 g
Fat: 15 g
Sugar: 5 g

INGREDIENTS

- 1 cup cooked wild rice (chilled or at room temperature)
- 1/2 cup cooked or canned chickpeas, roasted (optional)
- 1/2 cup chopped cucumber
- 1/4 cup Kalamata olives, sliced
- 2 tablespoons crumbled feta cheese
- 2 tablespoons lemon juice
- 1 tablespoon olive oil
- Pinch of salt
- Pinch of black pepper

INSTRUCTIONS

1. (Optional) Preheat your oven to 400°F (200°C). Spread chickpeas on a baking sheet. Drizzle with a small amount of olive oil, a pinch of salt, and a pinch of pepper. Roast for 15-20 minutes, or until golden brown and slightly crispy.

2. Wash and chop the cucumber into small, bite-sized pieces. Slice Kalamata olives in half lengthwise.

3. In a small bowl, whisk together lemon juice, olive oil, a pinch of salt, and a pinch of black pepper.

4. Combine the cooked wild rice, roasted chickpeas (if using), chopped cucumber, sliced olives, and crumbled feta cheese in a medium bowl.

5. Drizzle the lemon vinaigrette over the wild rice mixture. Gently toss to coat. Enjoy immediately.

SPICY BLACK BEAN BURRITO BOWL

SERVES: 2 • PREP TIME: 5 MIN • COOK TIME: 10 MIN

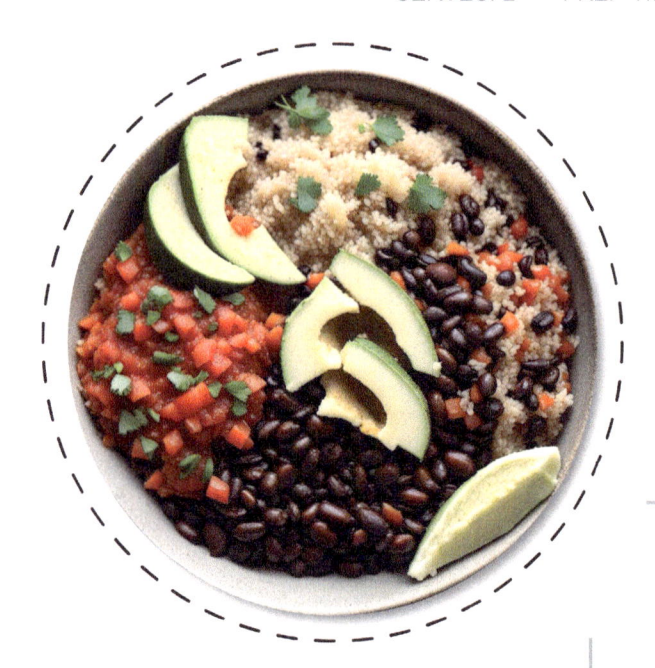

This Spicy Black Bean Burrito Bowl is a flavor-packed powerhouse of plant-based protein, fiber-rich brown rice, and creamy avocado. Get a vibrant kick from fire-roasted salsa and a squeeze of lime, while smoky chipotle spices add warmth and a metabolic boost. It's a satisfying and nutritious way to fuel your day!

NUTRITIONAL FACTS *(per serving)*

Calories: 350
Carbohydrates: 50g
Fiber: 12 g
Protein: 15 g
Fat: 12 g
Sugar: 5 g

INGREDIENTS

- 1 cup cooked brown rice
- 1 (15-ounce) can black beans, rinsed and drained
- 1/2 teaspoon chipotle chili powder
- 1/4 teaspoon cumin
- 1/4 teaspoon garlic powder
- 1/2 cup fire-roasted salsa
- 1/4 avocado, diced
- Squeeze of fresh lime juice
- Salt and pepper to taste

INSTRUCTIONS

1. Simmer the beans: In a medium saucepan, combine black beans, chipotle chili powder, cumin, garlic powder, and a splash of water or vegetable broth. Simmer over medium-low heat for 10-15 minutes, or until heated through and flavors meld.

2. Build your bowl: In a serving bowl, add a scoop of warm brown rice. Top with the seasoned black beans, a dollop of fire-roasted salsa, and diced avocado.

3. Flavor Boost: Squeeze fresh lime juice over the bowl and season with salt and pepper to taste.

CALIFORNIA-STYLE SUSHI ROLL

SERVES: 2 ROLLS • PREP TIME: 20 MIN • COOK TIME: 0 MIN

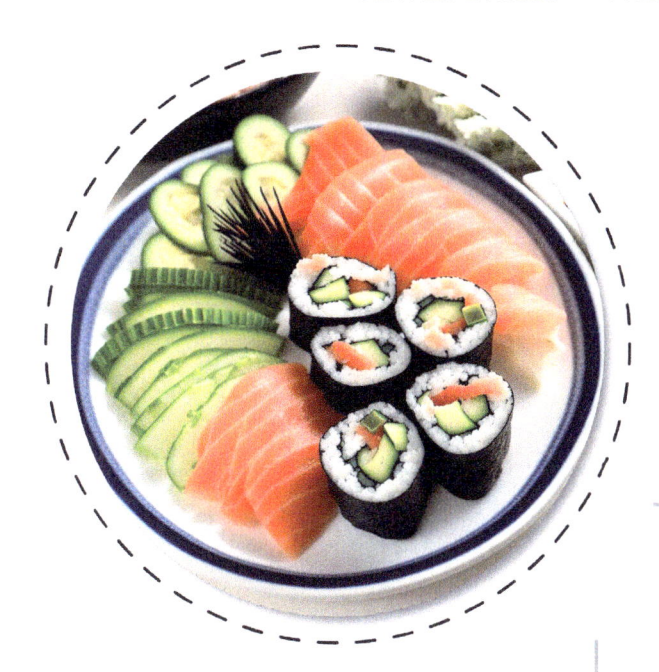

Homemade California-Style Sushi Rolls are a delicious and surprisingly easy culinary **adventure**! Enjoy the classic flavors of fresh avocado, cucumber, smoked salmon, and a hint of wasabi heat. Making your own sushi means you control the freshness, portions, and sodium levels – a healthy upgrade to your sushi night!

NUTRITIONAL FACTS *(per roll)*

Calories: 80
Carbohydrates: 10g
Fiber: 1 g
Protein: 3 g
Fat: 3 g
Sugar: 1 g

INGREDIENTS

- 1 cup cooked sushi rice (seasoned with rice vinegar, sugar, salt)
- 2 sheets nori seaweed
- 1/2 avocado, thinly sliced
- 1/4 cucumber, thinly sliced
- 3-4 ounces smoked salmon, thinly sliced
- Wasabi paste (optional)
- Soy sauce for serving

INSTRUCTIONS

1. Prep your ingredients: Cook sushi rice according to package directions. Season with rice vinegar, sugar, and salt mixture. Let cool slightly. Slice avocado, cucumber, and smoked salmon.

2. Assemble the rolls: Place a sheet of nori, shiny side down, on a bamboo sushi mat. Spread a thin, even layer of seasoned sushi rice over the nori, leaving a 1-inch border at the top. Arrange a line of avocado, cucumber, and salmon slices along the center of the rice. If desired, spread a very thin layer of wasabi paste over the fillings.

3. Roll it up: Starting from the end closest to you, gently lift the bamboo mat and begin rolling the sushi upwards, pressing gently to form a tight cylinder. Moisten the edge of the nori with water to seal the roll.

4. Cut and serve: Using a sharp knife, cut the sushi roll into 6-8 even pieces. Serve immediately with soy sauce and additional wasabi, if desired.

THAI CURRY CHICKEN BOWL

SERVES: 4 • PREP TIME: 15 MIN • COOK TIME: 30 MIN

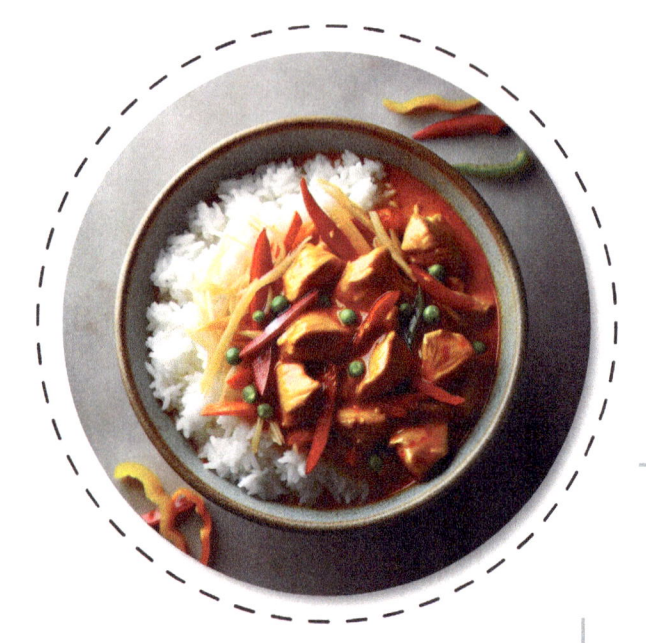

Experience Thailand in a bowl with this Thai Red Curry Chicken Bowl! Tender chicken and colorful vegetables simmer in a creamy, lightened-up red curry sauce infused with coconut milk and fragrant spices. Served over jasmine rice, it's a deliciously satisfying meal with a balance of protein, carbs, healthy fats, and vibrant flavors.

NUTRITIONAL FACTS *(per serving)*

Calories: 400　　**Protein**: 35 g
Carbohydrates: 35 g　　**Fat**: 15 g
Fiber: 5 g　　**Sugar**: 8 g

INGREDIENTS

- 1 cup cooked jasmine rice
- 1 tablespoon vegetable oil (or preferred cooking oil)
- 1 pound boneless, skinless chicken breast, diced
- 1/2 cup chopped onion
- 1/2 cup chopped bell pepper (any color)
- 2 tablespoons Thai red curry paste
- 1 (14-ounce) can light coconut milk
- 1 cup chicken broth (low-sodium)
- 1/2 cup bamboo shoots, sliced
- Salt and pepper to taste

INSTRUCTIONS

1. **Prep your ingredients**: Cook jasmine rice according to package directions (typically this involves simmering for 15-20 minutes). Dice the chicken breast, chop the onion and bell pepper, and slice the bamboo shoots if needed.

2. **Sauté the chicken**: Heat vegetable oil in a large skillet or wok over medium-high heat. Add diced chicken and cook for 5-7 minutes, or until browned on all sides and cooked through. Remove chicken and set aside.

3. **Build the flavor base**: In the same skillet, add onion and bell pepper. Sauté for 3-5 minutes, or until softened. Stir in the red curry paste and cook for 1 minute more, allowing the fragrance to bloom.

4. **Simmer the curry sauce**: Pour in light coconut milk and chicken broth. Bring to a gentle simmer. Add sliced bamboo shoots and return the cooked chicken to the pan. Reduce heat to low and simmer for 10-15 minutes, or until the sauce thickens slightly and chicken is heated through. Season with salt and pepper to taste.

5. **Assemble and enjoy**: Divide the warm jasmine rice into bowls. Top with the Thai red curry chicken and vegetables. Garnish with fresh cilantro (optional) and serve immediately.

LEMONY SHRIMP & WILD RICE

SERVES: 4   •   PREP TIME: 15 MIN   •   COOK TIME: 7 MIN

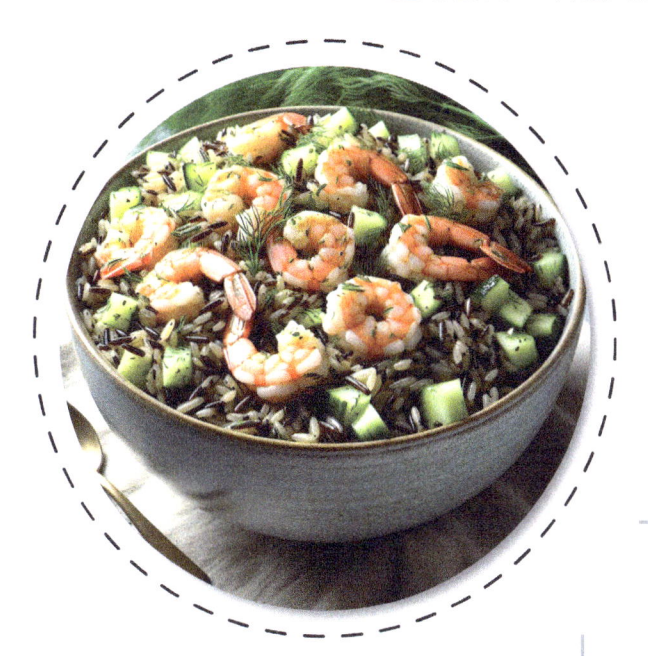

This Lemony Shrimp & Wild Rice Salad is a light and refreshing option packed with health benefits! Plump shrimp deliver lean protein for sustained energy, while wild rice provides fiber and complex carbohydrates for lasting satisfaction. Fresh dill and parsley add vibrant flavor and a boost of antioxidants to support overall health. A zesty lemon-olive oil dressing keeps it light and flavorful. It's a delicious and easy way to nourish your body!

NUTRITIONAL FACTS *(per serving)*

Calories: 300
Carbohydrates: 25 g
Fiber: 4 g
Protein: 28 g
Fat: 12 g
Sugar: 4 g

INGREDIENTS

- 1 cup cooked wild rice (chilled)
- 1 pound medium shrimp, peeled and deveined
- 1/4 cup chopped fresh dill
- 1/4 cup chopped fresh parsley
- 1/2 cup diced cucumber
- 3 tablespoons lemon juice
- 2 tablespoons olive oil
- 1/4 teaspoon salt
- 1/4 teaspoon black pepper

INSTRUCTIONS

1. Cook the shrimp: Bring a pot of salted water to a boil. Add the shrimp and cook for 2-3 minutes, or until they turn pink and are cooked through. Drain and rinse with cold water to stop the cooking process. Set aside to cool.

2. Prep the veggies and herbs: Wash and thoroughly dry the dill and parsley. Chop into small pieces. Dice the cucumber.

3. Make the dressing: In a small bowl, whisk together the lemon juice, olive oil, salt, and pepper, until well-combined.

4. Assemble the salad: In a large bowl, combine the cooked wild rice, cooled shrimp, chopped herbs, diced cucumber, and the lemon vinaigrette dressing. Gently toss to coat all ingredients evenly with the dressing.

5. Chill and serve: For the best flavor and texture, cover and refrigerate the salad for at least 30 minutes before serving. This allows the flavors to meld and the salad to chill. Serve cold or at room temperature.

VIETNAMESE PAPER ROLLS

SERVES: 7-8 ROLLS • PREP TIME: 20 MIN • COOK TIME: 0 MIN

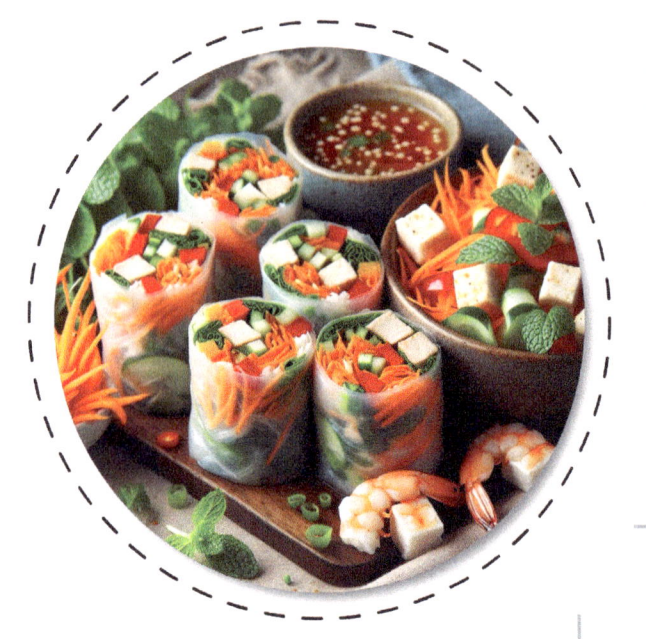

Vietnamese Rice Paper Rolls offer a light, refreshing, and incredibly flavorful culinary adventure! These delicate rolls star fresh vegetables, lean protein like grilled chicken or tofu, and fragrant herbs for a vibrant flavor burst. They're customizable to your taste and so satisfying despite being light and healthy. The interactive assembly and delicious sweet chili dipping sauce make them a fun and delicious choice for a nourishing meal!

NUTRITIONAL FACTS *(per roll)*

Calories: 100-150   **Protein**: 5-10 g
Carbohydrates: 15-20 g   **Fat**: 2-5 g
Fiber: 2-3 g   **Sugar**: 5 g

INGREDIENTS

- 8 sheets round rice paper
- 1 cup cooked and shredded protein (grilled chicken, baked tofu, shrimp)
- 1 cup assorted julienned vegetables (ex: carrots, bell peppers, cucumbers)
- 1/2 cup fresh mint leaves
- 1/4 cup fresh cilantro leaves (optional)
- Sweet chili dipping sauce for serving

INSTRUCTIONS

1. Prep your ingredients: Cook and shred your protein of choice – grilled chicken, baked tofu, or cooked shrimp all work well. Wash and julienne (cut into thin matchstick-size strips) vegetables like carrots, bell peppers, and cucumbers. Pick the leaves from fresh mint (and cilantro, if using).

2. Soften the rice paper: Fill a shallow dish or pie plate with warm water. Working with one at a time, dip a sheet of rice paper into the water for 5-10 seconds, just until softened and pliable. Don't oversoak!

3. Assemble the rolls: Lay the softened rice paper on a flat surface. Arrange a small pile of shredded protein, julienned vegetables, and a few herb leaves across the center of the rice paper. Fold the bottom of the rice paper up over the filling, then fold in the sides. Continue rolling tightly to form a cylinder.

4. Serve and enjoy: Repeat the process with the remaining rice paper and ingredients. Serve immediately with a side of sweet chili dipping sauce.

TUSCAN BROWN RICE & LENTIL SOUP

SERVES: 6-8 • PREP TIME: 15 MIN • COOK TIME: 50 MIN

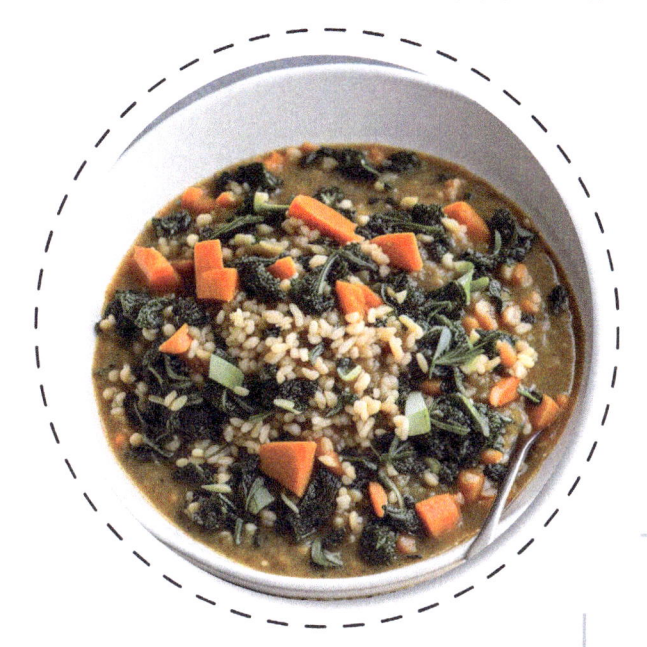

The hearty combination of protein-rich lentils, fiber-packed brown rice, and nutrient-dense Tuscan kale creates a powerhouse of nutrition. White wine and rosemary add a flavorful depth that makes this soup as delicious as it is good for you. It's a perfect choice for meal prepping and delivers a warm, comforting boost to your day.

NUTRITIONAL FACTS *(per serving)*

Calories: 250   **Protein**: 12 g
Carbohydrates: 35 g   **Fat**: 8 g
Fiber: 10 g   **Sugar**: 5 g

INGREDIENTS

- 1 tablespoon olive oil
- 1 medium onion, chopped
- 2 carrots, chopped
- 2 stalks celery, chopped
- 3 cloves garlic, minced
- 1 cup brown rice
- 1 cup green lentils, rinsed
- 6 cups vegetable broth
- 1/4 cup dry white wine
- 1 teaspoon dried rosemary
- 1 bunch Tuscan kale, stems removed, leaves roughly chopped
- Salt and pepper to taste

INSTRUCTIONS

1. Sauté the aromatics: Heat olive oil in a large pot or Dutch oven over medium heat. Add the chopped onion, carrots, and celery. Sauté for 5-7 minutes, or until vegetables soften. Stir in the minced garlic and cook for 1 minute more, until fragrant.

2. Add the main ingredients: Add the brown rice, lentils, vegetable broth, white wine, and dried rosemary to the pot. Bring to a boil, then reduce heat to low and cover.

3. Simmer for tenderness: Simmer for 30-40 minutes, or until the lentils and brown rice are tender. Stir occasionally to prevent sticking.

4. Incorporate the kale: Roughly chop the Tuscan kale leaves and stir them into the soup. Simmer for an additional 5-10 minutes, or until the kale wilts and softens.

5. Season and serve: Season the soup to taste with salt and black pepper. Serve hot, garnished with additional rosemary sprigs if desired.

MANGO SALSA RICE BOWL

SERVES: 4 • PREP TIME: 10 MIN • COOK TIME: 0 MIN

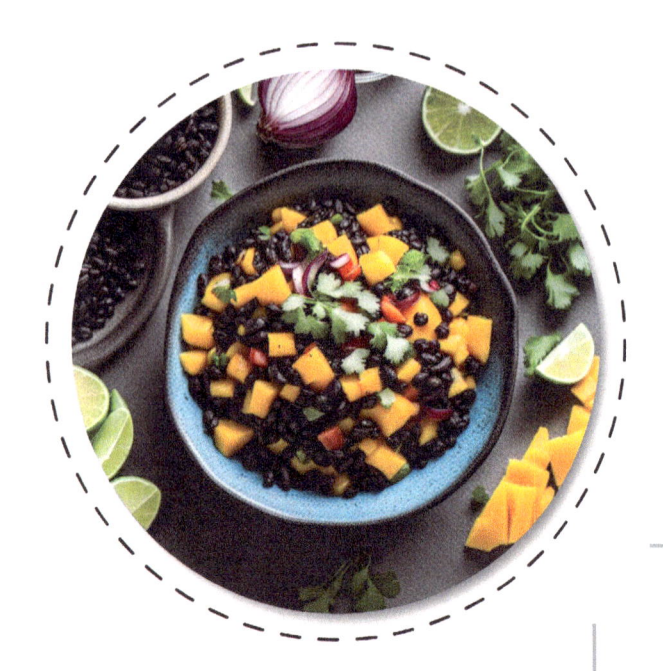

This Mango Salsa Rice Bowl is a delicious and nutritious burst of flavor! Earthy black rice and hearty black beans deliver a powerful dose of fiber, while mango, avocado, and cilantro pack in vitamins, minerals, and antioxidants. The lime juice and red onion add a zesty kick, creating a perfectly balanced and naturally filling meal. It's a healthy and vibrant way to fuel your day!

NUTRITIONAL FACTS *(per serving)*

Calories: 350

Carbohydrates: 50 g

Fiber: 15 g

Protein: 12 g

Fat: 15 g

Sugar: 10 g

INGREDIENTS

- 1 cup cooked black rice
- 1 (15-ounce) can black beans, rinsed and drained
- 1 large ripe mango, diced
- 1/2 avocado, diced
- 1/4 cup diced red onion
- 1/4 cup chopped fresh cilantro
- 2 tablespoons fresh lime juice
- Salt and pepper to taste

INSTRUCTIONS

1. Prepare the ingredients: Cook black rice according to package directions – typically, it involves simmering it for around 30 minutes. Dice the ripe mango, avocado, and red onion. Roughly chop the fresh cilantro.

2. Assemble the bowl: In a large bowl, combine the cooked black rice, black beans, diced mango, avocado, red onion, and chopped cilantro. Drizzle with fresh lime juice and season generously with salt and pepper. Gently toss to combine all the ingredients, ensuring everything is evenly coated with the lime juice and seasoning.

3. Serve and enjoy: Divide the mango salsa rice mixture into bowls and serve immediately for the best texture and vibrant flavors.

SPANISH-STYLE PAELLA

SERVES: 4 • PREP TIME: 20 MIN • COOK TIME: 35 MIN

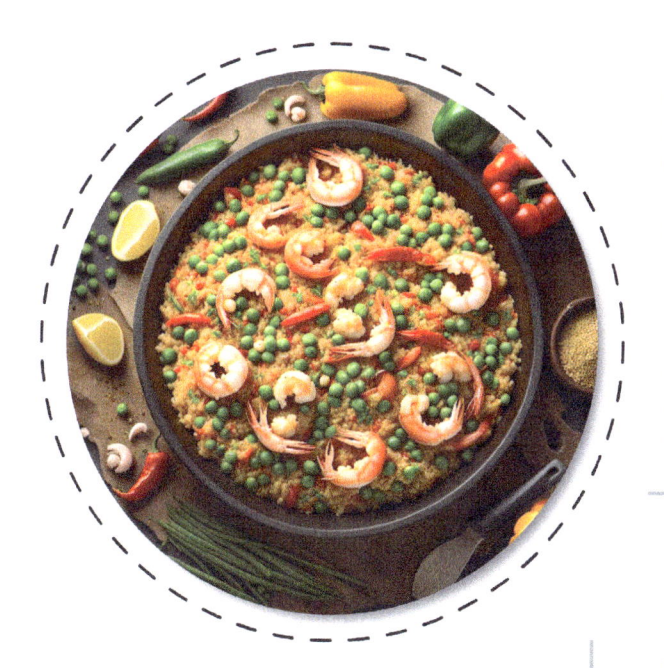

Enjoy the flavors of Spain with this healthier take on classic Spanish-Style Paella! The mix of nutty brown rice and cauliflower rice lowers carbs and calories while boosting the veggie content. Tender chicken, plump shrimp, and vibrant vegetables deliver satisfying lean protein and a burst of fresh flavor. Saffron adds its signature touch for an authentic and delicious experience!

NUTRITIONAL FACTS *(per serving)*

Calories: 350 **Protein**: 30 g
Carbohydrates: 30 g **Fat**: 12 g
Fiber: 6 g **Sugar**: 5 g

INGREDIENTS

- 1 tablespoon olive oil
- 1 pound boneless, skinless chicken thighs, cut into 1-inch pieces
- 1/2 pound medium shrimp, peeled and deveined
- 1/2 onion, chopped
- 1 bell pepper (any color), chopped
- 2 cloves garlic, minced
- 1 teaspoon smoked paprika
- Pinch of saffron threads
- 1 cup brown rice
- 1 cup cauliflower rice
- 2 cups chicken (or vegetable) broth
- 1/2 cup frozen peas
- Salt and pepper

INSTRUCTIONS

1. Heat olive oil in a large, wide skillet or paella pan over medium-high heat. Add chicken pieces and cook, stirring occasionally, until browned on all sides. Remove the chicken and set aside.

2. Add the shrimp to the same pan and cook for 2-3 minutes per side, or until pink and cooked through. Remove the shrimp and set aside.

3. Add onion and bell pepper to the pan, sauté for 5-7 minutes, or until softened. Stir in minced garlic and cook for 1 minute more.

4. Add smoked paprika and saffron threads to the pan, cook for 30 seconds, stirring constantly to release their aroma.

5. Stir the brown rice and cauliflower rice into the pan. Pour in the chicken broth. Season with salt and pepper. Bring to a simmer.

6. Reduce heat to low, cover, and simmer for 15-20 minutes, or until the rice is tender and most of the liquid is absorbed. Stir in the frozen peas, cooked chicken, and shrimp. Heat through for 2-3 minutes. Serve immediately, garnished with chopped parsley (optional) for a touch of freshness.

Speedy and Satisfying SNACKS

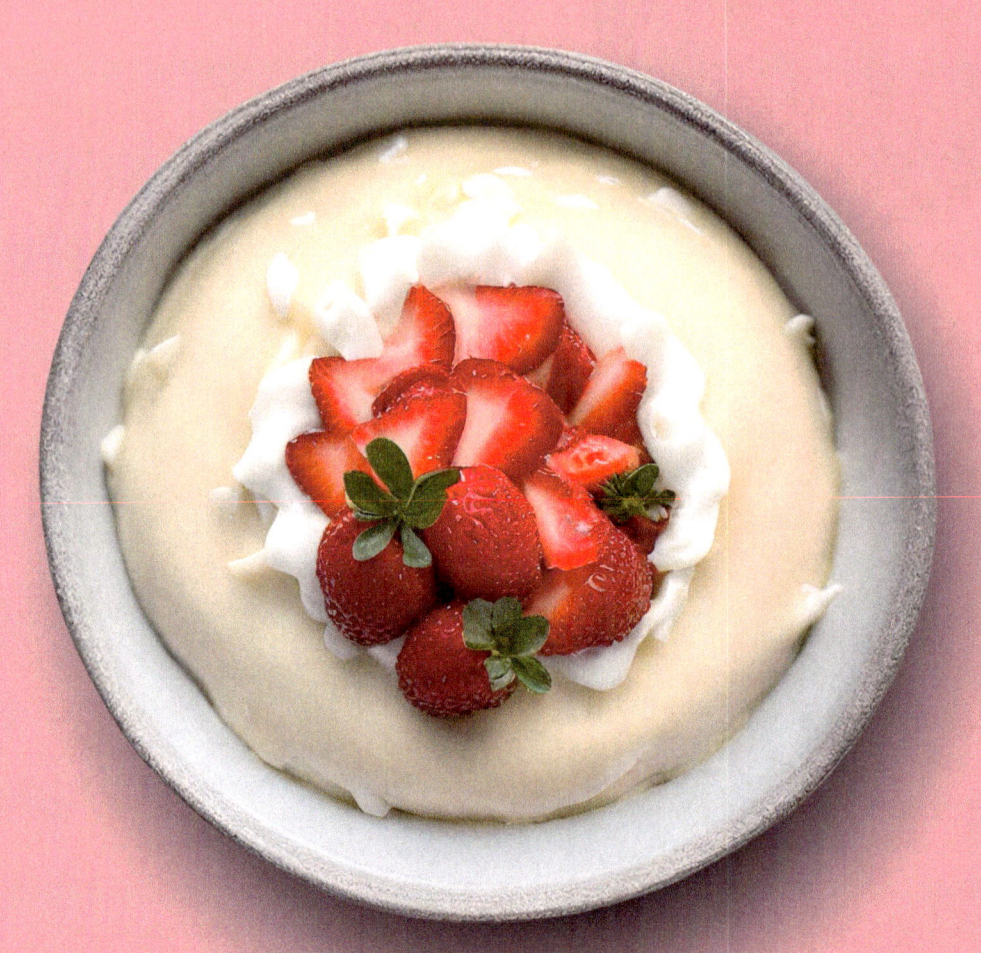

Forget the mid-day energy slumps! Smart snacking is key to a healthy diet, and we're ditching processed junk for something better – rice! The Exotic Rice Hack Diet is all about culinary adventure, and that includes snacks. From nutty forbidden rice to sweet jasmine, there's a world of flavors to discover. Think beyond meals – rice transforms into amazing finger foods, crackers, and treats! We'll show you how to make protein-packed snacks for lasting energy and fiber-rich options to keep you full. Say goodbye to chips and hello to global snacking excitement! Get ready to power through your day with delicious, healthy, and satisfying rice-based snacks.

CRISPY WILD RICE CRACKERS

SERVES: 4 • PREP TIME: 5 MIN • COOK TIME: 25 MIN

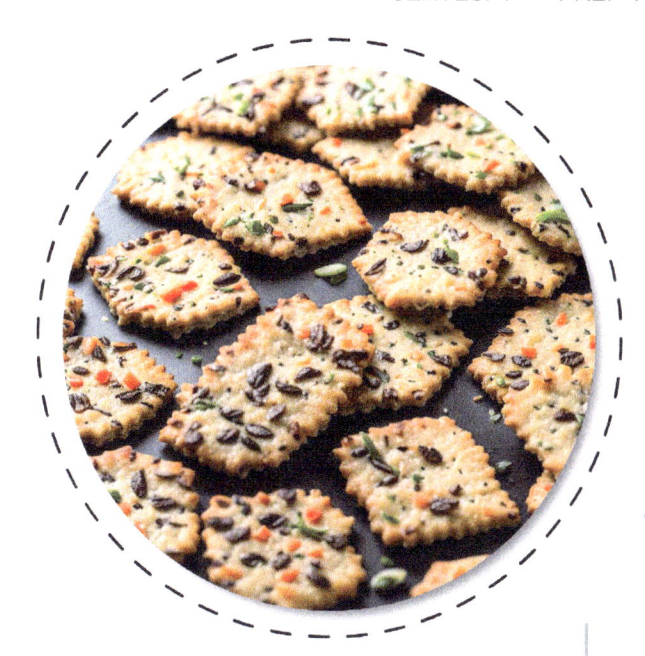

Get ready for a satisfyingly crunchy snack that's surprisingly easy to make and packed with the goodness of wild rice! These Crackers are a healthier alternative to processed crackers, offering a boost of fiber and a unique nutty flavor. Customize them with your favorite herbs and spices, and enjoy them with dips, cheese, or healthy toppings for a guilt-free snack that supports your weight loss goals.

NUTRITIONAL FACTS *(per serving)*

Calories: 120
Carbohydrates: 15 g
Fiber: 2 g
Protein: 3 g
Fat: 6 g
Sugar: 1 g

INGREDIENTS

- 1 cup cooked wild rice
- 1 tablespoon olive oil (or preferred oil)
- 1 teaspoon dried herbs (Italian seasoning, herbs de Provence, etc.)
- 1/2 teaspoon garlic powder
- 1/4 teaspoon salt
- 1/4 teaspoon black pepper

INSTRUCTIONS

1. Preheat your oven to 350°F (175°C) and line a baking sheet with parchment paper.

2. In a medium bowl, combine cooked wild rice, olive oil, herbs, garlic powder, salt, and pepper. Stir gently to coat the rice evenly.

3. Spread the seasoned wild rice mixture in a very thin, even layer onto the prepared baking sheet. The thinner the layer, the crispier your crackers will be.

4. Bake for 20-25 minutes, or until the edges are lightly browned and the crackers feel dry and crispy to the touch.

5. Allow the crackers to cool completely on the baking sheet. Once cooled, break them into irregular pieces.

6. Store crispy rice crackers in an airtight container at room temperature for up to a week. Enjoy as a base for spreads, with dips, or on their own!

MEDITERRANEAN RICE BALLS

SERVES: 12-14 RICE BALLS • PREP TIME: 10 MIN • COOK TIME: 20 MIN

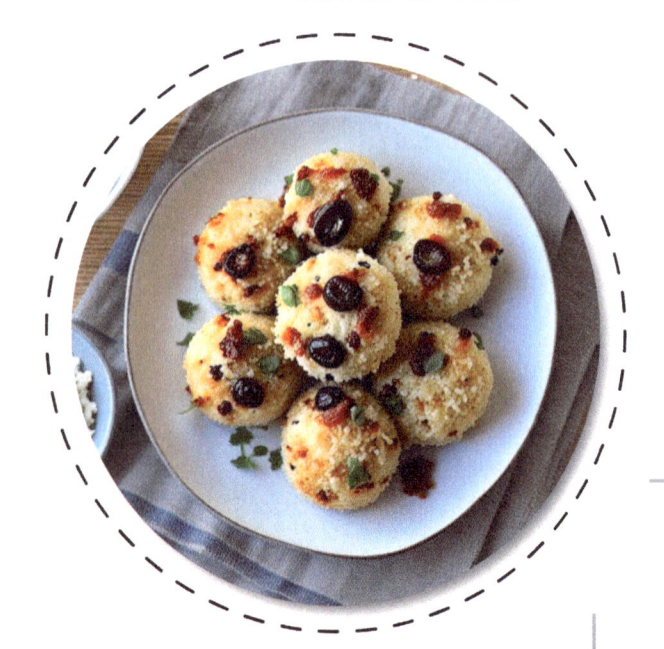

This recipe is the perfect snack for healthy and flavorful satisfaction! Basmati rice, olives, sun-dried tomatoes, feta, and herbs combine for a delicious burst of flavor. They offer a balanced mix of carbs and healthy fats for lasting energy. Plus, they're easy to make ahead for grab-and-go convenience!

NUTRITIONAL FACTS *(per rice ball)*

Calories: 80
Carbohydrates: 9 g
Fiber: 1 g
Protein: 2 g
Fat: 4 g
Sugar: 1 g

INGREDIENTS

- 1 cup cooked basmati rice (chilled or at room temperature)
- 1/4 cup chopped Kalamata olives
- 1/4 cup chopped sun-dried tomatoes
- 1/4 cup crumbled feta cheese
- 2 tablespoons chopped fresh parsley (or other herbs like oregano and basil)
- 1 tablespoon olive oil
- Pinch of salt
- Pinch of black pepper

INSTRUCTIONS

1. In a medium bowl, combine the cooked basmati rice, chopped olives, sun-dried tomatoes, crumbled feta cheese, chopped parsley, olive oil, salt, and pepper. Mix gently until evenly combined.

2. Form the rice balls: Shape the rice mixture into small, bite-sized balls (approximately 1-inch in diameter).

3. Preheat your oven to 400°F (200°C). Line a baking sheet with parchment paper (optional) or lightly grease the pan. Place the rice balls on the prepared baking sheet and bake for 15-20 minutes, or until lightly golden brown and heated through.

4. Serve and enjoy: Serve the rice balls warm for the best texture and flavor. They can also be enjoyed at room temperature.

THAI COCONUT RICE PUDDING BITES

SERVES: 4-6 • PREP TIME: 5 MIN • COOK TIME: 0 MIN

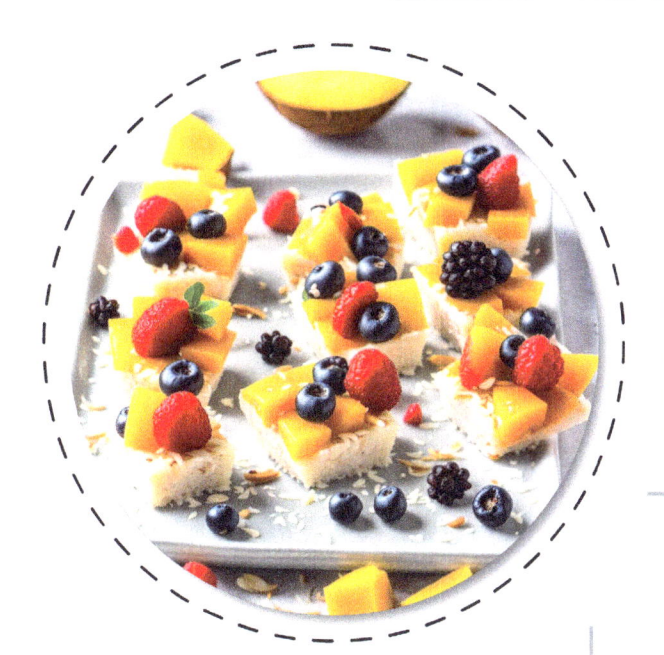

This pudding transport you to Thailand with their light, refreshing flavor! Fragrant jasmine rice, creamy coconut milk, and a hint of sweetness create perfectly portioned treats for a satisfying, not overly indulgent, snack. They're easy to make ahead, delivering a taste of creamy, tropical goodness whenever a craving hits.

NUTRITIONAL FACTS *(per serving)*

Calories: 120 **Protein:** 2 g
Carbohydrates: 20 g **Fat:** 5 g
Fiber: 1 g **Sugar:** 8 g

INGREDIENTS

- 1 cup cooked jasmine rice (chilled)
- 1/2 cup full-fat coconut milk
- 1 tablespoon maple syrup (or honey, or your preferred sweetener)
- 1/2 teaspoon vanilla extract
- Pinch of salt
- Toppings (optional): toasted coconut flakes, fresh berries, chopped mango

INSTRUCTIONS

1. In a blender or food processor, combine the chilled cooked jasmine rice, coconut milk, maple syrup (or preferred sweetener), vanilla extract, and a pinch of salt. Blend until smooth and creamy.

2. Portion and chill: Divide the rice pudding mixture evenly into small serving cups or ramekins. Cover and refrigerate for at least 2 hours, or ideally overnight, to allow the flavors to meld and the pudding to set.

3. Just before serving, top with your desired toppings (optional), such as toasted coconut flakes, fresh berries, or chopped mango for an extra burst of flavor and texture. Enjoy cold!

SAVORY SUSHI MUFFINS

SERVES: 12 MUFFINS • PREP TIME: 10 MIN • COOK TIME: 25 MIN

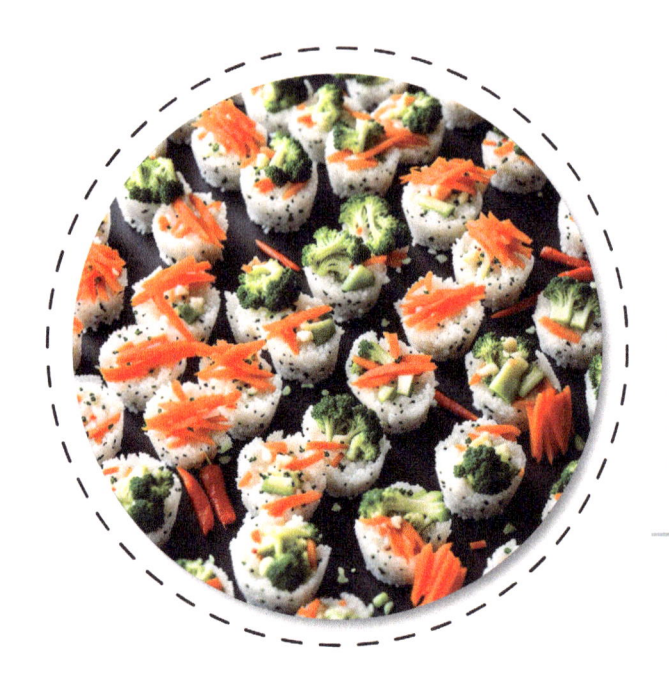

Savory Sushi Rice Muffins are a smart and delicious way to use up leftover sushi rice! They're a balanced snack with protein, carbs, and veggies for sustained energy and essential nutrients. They're perfect for preventing food waste and offer endless customization with different veggies or added protein. Plus, you can freeze them for healthy grab-and-go bites anytime!

NUTRITIONAL FACTS *(per serving)*

Calories: 120 **Protein**: 4 g
Carbohydrates: 18 g **Fat**: 4 g
Fiber: 2 g **Sugar**: 2 g

INGREDIENTS

- 2 cups cooked sushi rice
- 1/2 cup chopped mixed vegetables (carrots, bell peppers, broccoli, etc.)
- 1 large egg
- 1 tablespoon soy sauce (or use low-sodium soy sauce)
- 1 teaspoon sesame oil (optional)
- Optional: sesame seeds, green onions, sriracha sauce (for serving)

INSTRUCTIONS

1. Preheat your oven to 375°F (190°C). Grease a standard 12-cup muffin tin or use muffin liners.

2. In a large bowl, combine the cooked sushi rice, chopped vegetables, egg, soy sauce, and sesame oil (if using). Mix well until all ingredients are evenly combined.

3. Fill the muffin tin: Divide the rice mixture evenly among the prepared muffin cups, filling them about 2/3 of the way full.

4. Bake the muffins: Bake for 20-25 minutes, or until the muffins are set and lightly golden brown on top.

5. Let the muffins cool slightly in the pan before removing. Serve warm or at room temperature. Top with sesame seeds, sliced green onions, or your favorite sauce (like sriracha) if desired.

SWEET & SALTY BLACK RICE MIX

SERVES: 2-3 • PREP TIME: 15 MIN • COOK TIME: 7 MIN

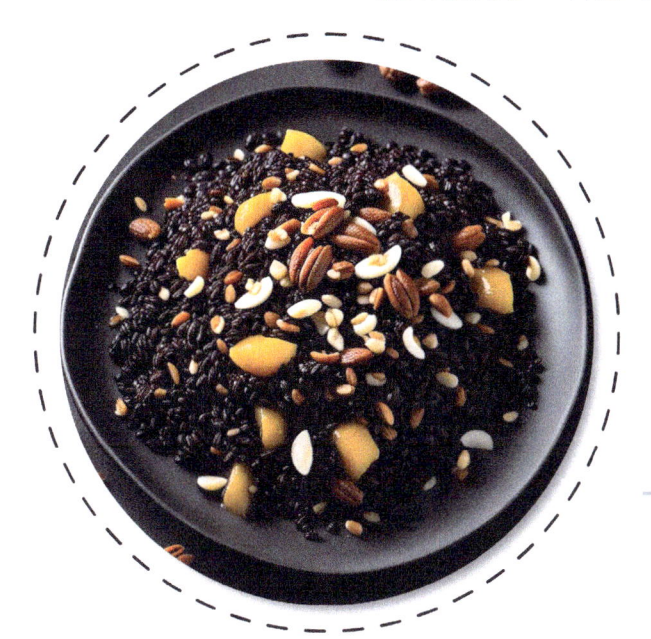

This snack is a delicious way to fuel your body! Puffed black rice delivers fiber and antioxidants, while toasted nuts offer a satisfying boost of protein and healthy fats. The light touch of sweetness makes it a perfectly balanced snack to curb cravings while nourishing your body.

NUTRITIONAL FACTS *(per serving)*

Calories: 200 **Protein**: 5 g
Carbohydrates: 20 g **Fat**: 10 g
Fiber: 2 g **Sugar**: 8 g

INGREDIENTS

- 1 cup puffed black rice
- 1/2 cup mixed toasted nuts (almonds, cashews, pecans, etc.)
- 1 tablespoon pure maple syrup (or honey)
- 1/2 teaspoon vanilla extract (optional)
- Pinch of sea salt
- Pinch of ground cinnamon (optional)

INSTRUCTIONS

1. Toast the nuts (optional): If using raw nuts, preheat your oven to 350°F (175°C). Spread the nuts on a baking sheet lined with parchment paper and toast for 5-7 minutes, or until fragrant and lightly golden brown. Let them cool completely before using.

2. Combine the ingredients: In a large bowl, combine the puffed black rice and toasted nuts.

3. Make the sweet and salty drizzle: In a small bowl, whisk together the maple syrup (or honey), vanilla extract (if using), sea salt, and ground cinnamon (if using).

4. Pour the sweet and salty drizzle over the rice and nut mixture. Use a spoon or spatula to gently toss and coat everything evenly.

5. (Optional) For a slightly more clustered snack mix, spread the coated mixture on a baking sheet lined with parchment paper and let it sit for 10-15 minutes, allowing the drizzle to harden slightly.

6. Break it up and enjoy! Once set (if desired), break up any large clumps and enjoy your sweet and salty black rice snack mix!

KOREAN KIMCHI RICE CAKES

SERVES: 4-6 RICE CAKES • PREP TIME: 5 MIN • COOK TIME: 12 MIN

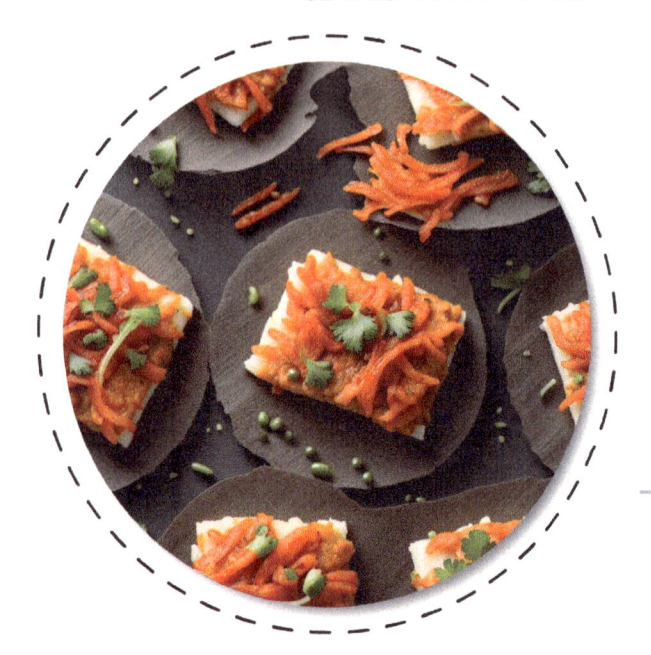

Korean Kimchi Rice Cakes are a unique and satisfying snack! The fermented kimchi delivers gut-friendly probiotics for digestive and overall health. Crispy pan-fried rice creates the perfect base for the kimchi's tangy, spicy flavor. It's a quick and easy way to enjoy classic Korean flavors and boost your gut health all at once.

NUTRITIONAL FACTS *(per serving)*

Calories: 200
Carbohydrates: 20 g
Fiber: 2 g
Protein: 5 g
Fat: 10 g
Sugar: 8 g

INGREDIENTS

- 1 cup cooked short-grain rice (sushi rice is ideal)
- 2-3 tablespoons vegetable oil (or preferred cooking oil)
- 1/2 cup kimchi, roughly chopped
- Toppings (optional): sliced green onions, toasted sesame seeds

INSTRUCTIONS

1. Shape the cooked rice into small, flat patties (about 1/2 inch thick). You can do this using your hands or a small round cookie cutter for more uniform shapes.

2. Heat 1 tablespoon of vegetable oil in a large non-stick skillet over medium-high heat.

3. Place the rice cakes in the hot skillet, working in batches if needed to avoid overcrowding the pan. Cook for 3-4 minutes per side, or until golden brown and crispy. Add more oil to the pan as needed.

4. Place the crispy rice cakes on a serving plate. Top each rice cake with a dollop of kimchi. Garnish with sliced green onions and toasted sesame seeds (optional). Serve warm and enjoy immediately for the best texture!

TROPICAL FRUIT & RICE SALAD CUPS

SERVES: 4-6 • PREP TIME: 10 MIN • COOK TIME: 0 MIN

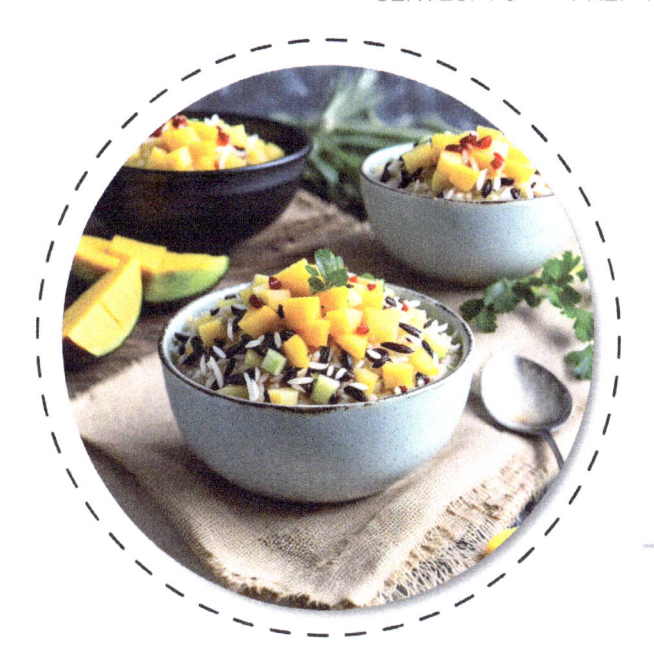

Escape to the tropics with these vibrant recipe! Wild rice delivers fiber and satisfying texture, while mango and pineapple burst with natural sweetness, vitamins, and antioxidants. Toasted coconut adds a healthy fat boost and nutty flavor. These refreshing cups are perfect for hydrating and nourishing your body on the go.

NUTRITIONAL FACTS *(per serving)*

Calories: 150   **Protein**: 2 g
Carbohydrates: 30 g **Fat**: 3 g
Fiber: 3 g   **Sugar**: 15 g

INGREDIENTS

- 1 cup cooked wild rice (chilled)
- 1 cup diced mango
- 1/2 cup diced pineapple
- 1-2 tablespoons toasted coconut flakes
- Optional: Squeeze of fresh lime juice

INSTRUCTIONS

1. Prep the fruit: Dice the mango and pineapple into small, bite-sized pieces.

2. Toast the coconut flakes (optional): Heat a small skillet over medium-low heat. Add coconut flakes and toast for 2-3 minutes, or until lightly golden brown and fragrant. Let them cool completely before using.

3. Assemble the cups: In each serving cup or ramekin, layer the ingredients. Start with a layer of chilled wild rice, then add the diced mango and pineapple.

4. Top and serve: Sprinkle each cup with a generous amount of toasted coconut flakes. If desired, add a light squeeze of lime juice for a touch of citrusy brightness. Serve chilled and enjoy!

CHINESE RED RICE "POPCORN"

SERVES: 2-3 • PREP TIME: 5 MIN • COOK TIME: 7 MIN

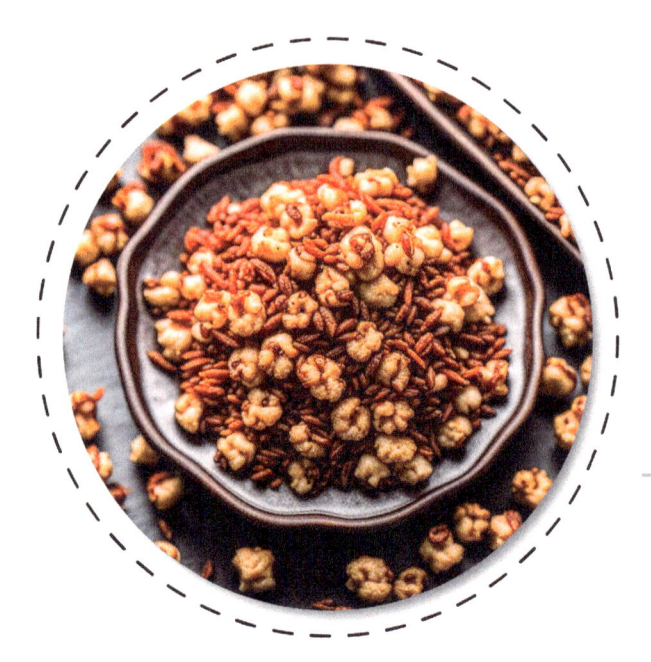

Chinese Red Rice "Popcorn" is a delicious and healthy way to satisfy snack cravings! This whole-grain alternative offers fiber, a nutty flavor, and a satisfying crunch. Customize it with your favorite herbs and spices for a light, airy snack that's both fun to make and good for you.

NUTRITIONAL FACTS *(per serving)*

Calories: 150	**Protein**: 3 g
Carbohydrates: 25 g	**Fat**: 4 g
Fiber: 2 g	**Sugar**: 1 g

INGREDIENTS

- 1/2 cup red rice kernels
- 1 tablespoon olive oil (or preferred cooking oil)
- Pinch of salt
- Desired Herbs (optional): Italian seasoning, rosemary, garlic powder, chili powder, etc.

INSTRUCTIONS

1. Heat the olive oil in a large pot with a tight-fitting lid over medium heat.

2. Once the oil is hot, carefully add the red rice kernels to the pot in a single layer. It's important not to overcrowd the pot.

3. Reduce the heat to medium-low and immediately cover the pot with the tight-fitting lid. Listen for the popping sounds as the kernels start to explode.

4. While the kernels are popping, gently shake the pot occasionally to prevent burning. Do not lift the lid to peek, as this can release steam and prevent popping.

5. Once the popping sounds become infrequent, with pauses of several seconds between pops, remove the pot from the heat. This indicates that most of the kernels have popped.

6. Carefully open the pot away from your face to release any steam. Transfer the popped red rice to a bowl and season with a pinch of salt. Sprinkle with your desired herbs (optional) and toss to coat. Enjoy immediately for the best texture!

ITALIAN RICE PUDDING PARFAIT

SERVES: 2-4 • PREP TIME: 10 MIN • COOK TIME: 0 MIN

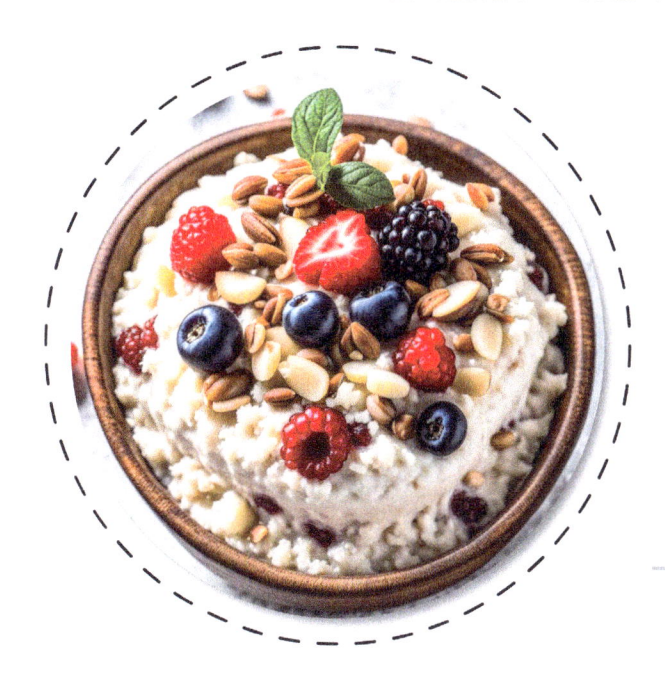

This recipe is a satisfying and nourishing treat perfect for mindful indulgence. Creamy arborio rice and low-fat ricotta create a protein-rich base, while honey adds natural sweetness. Cinnamon adds warmth, and the individual portions help control intake. It's the perfect way to satisfy your sweet tooth while staying on track with your health goals.

NUTRITIONAL FACTS *(per serving)*

Calories: 150   **Protein**: 10 g
Carbohydrates: 20 g   **Fat**: 4 g
Fiber: 1 g   **Sugar**: 10 g

INGREDIENTS

- 1 cup cooked arborio rice (chilled)
- 1/2 cup low-fat ricotta cheese
- 1 tablespoon honey
- 1/4 teaspoon ground cinnamon
- Optional Toppings: fresh berries, chopped nuts, cocoa nibs

INSTRUCTIONS

1. In a small bowl, whisk together the ricotta cheese, honey, and cinnamon until well combined and smooth.

2. In each serving glass or ramekin, layer the ingredients. Start with a layer of chilled, cooked arborio rice, followed by a generous dollop of the ricotta cheese mixture. Repeat the layering once more.

3. Top each parfait with your desired toppings (if using). Some suggestions include fresh berries, chopped nuts, or a sprinkle of cocoa nibs. Serve immediately or chill until ready to enjoy.

SPICED BLACK RICE CRACKERS

SERVES: 20-25 CRACKERS • PREP TIME: 15 MIN • COOK TIME: 20-25 MIN

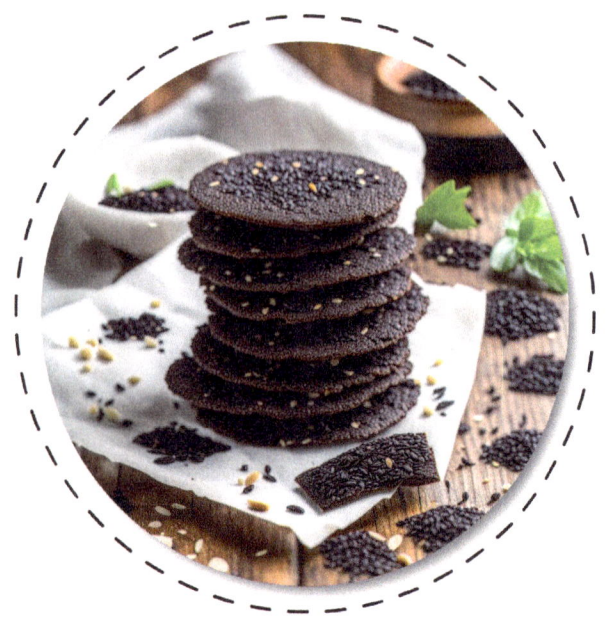

These Spiced Black Rice Crackers are the perfect way to upgrade your snacking! Black rice delivers fiber, antioxidants, and minerals, while flaxseed boosts omega-3 fatty acids and fiber for gut health. They're naturally gluten-free and customizable with your favorite spices for a delicious and nourishing crunch.

NUTRITIONAL FACTS *(per serving)*

Calories: 30
Carbohydrates: 5 g
Fiber: 1 g
Protein: 1 g
Fat: 1 g
Sugar: 1 g

INGREDIENTS

- 1 cup cooked black rice (cooled slightly)
- 1/4 cup ground flaxseed
- 1 teaspoon ground cumin
- 1/2 teaspoon ground coriander
- 1/4 teaspoon garlic powder
- Pinch of salt
- 1-2 tablespoons water (as needed)

INSTRUCTIONS

1. Grind the cooked black rice in a blender or food processor until it resembles a coarse flour. This step is optional, but it helps create a smoother cracker dough.
2. In a large bowl, combine the black rice, ground flaxseed, cumin, coriander, garlic powder, and salt. Mix well to distribute the spices evenly.
3. Slowly add water, 1 tablespoon at a time, and mix until a dough forms that is slightly sticky but holds its shape. You may not need all the water.
4. Preheat your oven to 350°F (175°C). Line a baking sheet with parchment paper.
5. Divide the dough in half. Place one half between two sheets of parchment paper. Use a rolling pin to roll out the dough into a thin sheet, aiming for about 1/8 inch thickness. Repeat with the other half of the dough on a separate parchment paper sheet.
6. Use a knife or cookie cutter to cut the rolled-out dough into desired shapes (squares, triangles, circles, etc.).
7. Transfer the parchment paper with the shaped dough onto the prepared baking sheet. Bake for 20-25 minutes, or until the crackers are golden brown and crisp around the edges.
8. Let the crackers cool completely on the baking sheet before transferring them to an airtight container.

PEANUT BUTTER BANANA RICE BITES

SERVES: 10-12 BITES • PREP TIME: 10 MIN • COOK TIME: 0 MIN

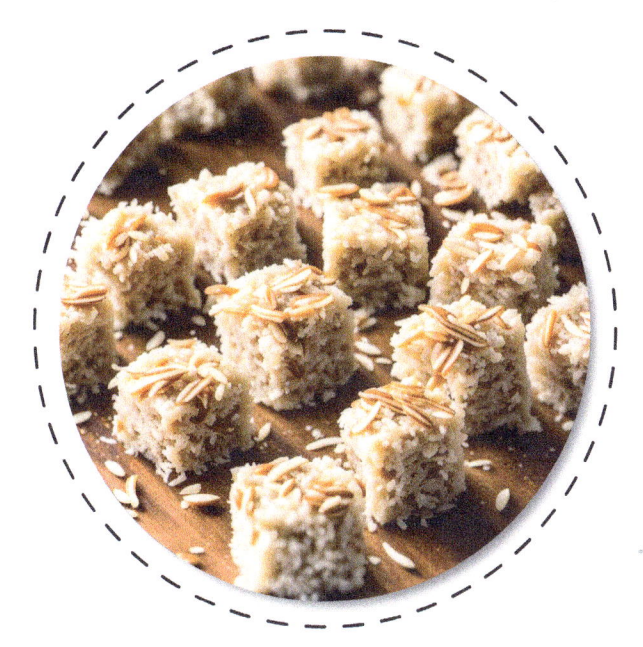

Fuel your day with Peanut Butter Banana Rice Bites! Creamy peanut butter and hearty brown rice deliver protein and fiber for lasting energy, while banana adds natural sweetness. A sprinkle of unsweetened coconut offers a taste of the tropics. These easy-to-make bites are a healthy, portable, and customizable way to beat snack cravings.

NUTRITIONAL FACTS *(per serving)*

Calories: 80
Carbohydrates: 10 g
Fiber: 2 g
Protein: 2 g
Fat: 4 g
Sugar: 5 g

INGREDIENTS

- 1 ripe banana, mashed
- 1/2 cup cooked brown rice (chilled)
- 2 tablespoons peanut butter (or preferred nut butter)
- 1/4 cup unsweetened shredded coconut)

INSTRUCTIONS

1. Add the chilled cooked brown rice and peanut butter. Mix well until thoroughly combined.

2. Shape the mixture into bite-sized balls (approximately 1 inch in diameter). You can slightly wet your hands to help prevent sticking.

3. Place unsweetened shredded coconut in a shallow dish or bowl. Gently roll each rice bite in the coconut, ensuring an even coating.

4. Chill and enjoy (optional): Place the coated bites on a baking sheet lined with parchment paper (optional) and chill in the refrigerator for 15-20 minutes for a firmer texture, if desired. Enjoy!

Dinner
DELIGHTS

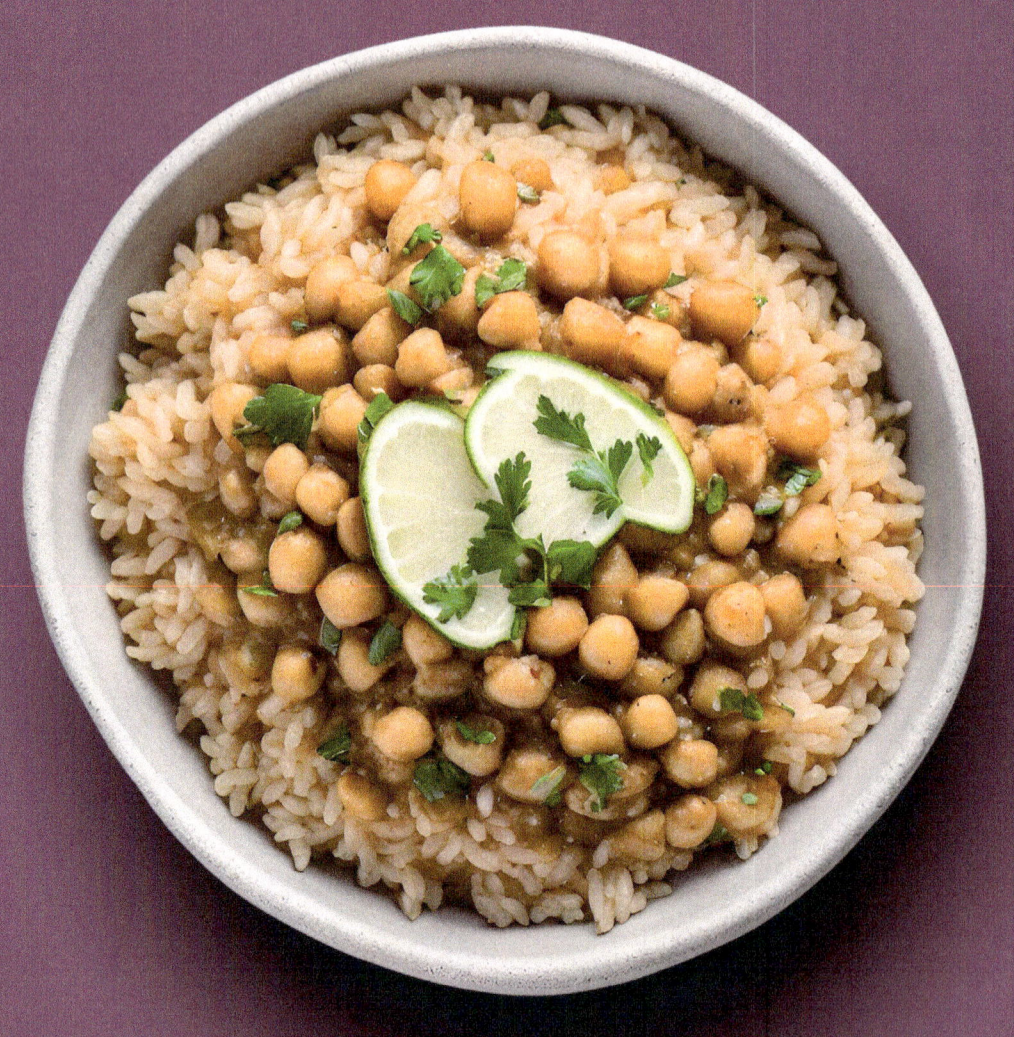

Let's dive into global recipes, healthy twists on classics, and perfect cooking techniques. Imagine vibrant stir-fries with earthy forbidden rice, nourishing grain bowls with fluffy Bhutanese red, or a fragrant Indian biryani with aromatic basmati. Exotic rice is your ticket to new techniques and flavors. Whether you're an experienced cook or a beginner, these grains will inspire you. Get ready to transform dinner into a global adventure filled with vibrant colors, textures, and incredible flavor!

SPANISH PAELLA REMIX

SERVES: 4-6 • PREP TIME: 15 MIN • COOK TIME: 30-35 MIN

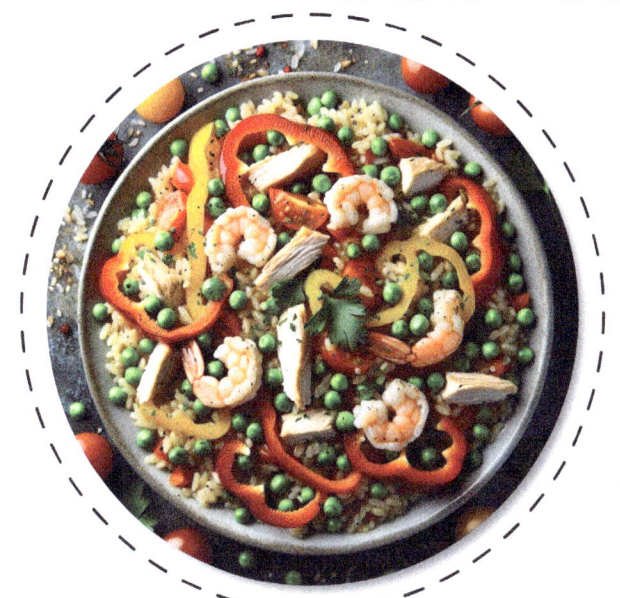

Enjoy a healthier, lighter take on classic paella! Brown rice and cauliflower rice offer fiber and nutrients while reducing carbs. Chicken and shrimp deliver satisfying protein, while a saffron-infused broth adds incredible flavor. It's a delicious and balanced way to experience this iconic dish.

NUTRITIONAL FACTS *(per serving)*

Calories: 350   **Protein**: 30 g
Carbohydrates: 35 g   **Fat**: 12 g
Fiber: 6 g   **Sugar**: 5 g

INGREDIENTS

- 1 cup cooked brown rice
- 1 cup cooked cauliflower rice
- 4 cups chicken broth (low-sodium preferred)
- 1/2 teaspoon ground saffron
- 1 tablespoon olive oil
- 1 medium onion, chopped
- 1 bell pepper, chopped (any color)
- 2 cloves garlic, minced
- 1 boneless, skinless chicken breast, cooked and shredded (about 1 cup)
- 1 cup peeled and deveined shrimp
- 1 cup frozen peas
- 1/2 cup chopped cherry tomatoes
- 1/4 cup chopped fresh parsley
- Salt and freshly ground black pepper to taste

INSTRUCTIONS

1. In a saucepan, heat the chicken broth over medium heat. Add the saffron and simmer for 5 minutes, allowing the flavors to infuse. Keep the broth warm.

2. Heat olive oil in a large skillet or paella pan over medium heat. Add the chopped onion and bell pepper. Sauté for 5-7 minutes, or until softened. Add the minced garlic and cook for an additional minute until fragrant.

3. Stir in the cooked brown rice and cauliflower rice. Pour in the warm saffron-infused chicken broth and bring to a simmer. Season with a pinch of salt and pepper.

4. Reduce heat to low, cover the pan, and simmer for 15 minutes, or until the rice is nearly cooked through and most of the broth has been absorbed. Nestle the cooked and shredded chicken and shrimp on top of the rice.

5. Gently stir in the frozen peas and cherry tomatoes. Cover the pan and cook for an additional 5 minutes, or until the shrimp are cooked through and the vegetables are heated.

6. Remove the pan from heat and let it stand for 5 minutes before serving. Garnish with chopped fresh parsley and enjoy immediately.

CHICKEN FAJITA BOWL

SERVES: 4 • PREP TIME: 20 MIN + MARINATING TIME • COOK TIME: 20-25 MIN

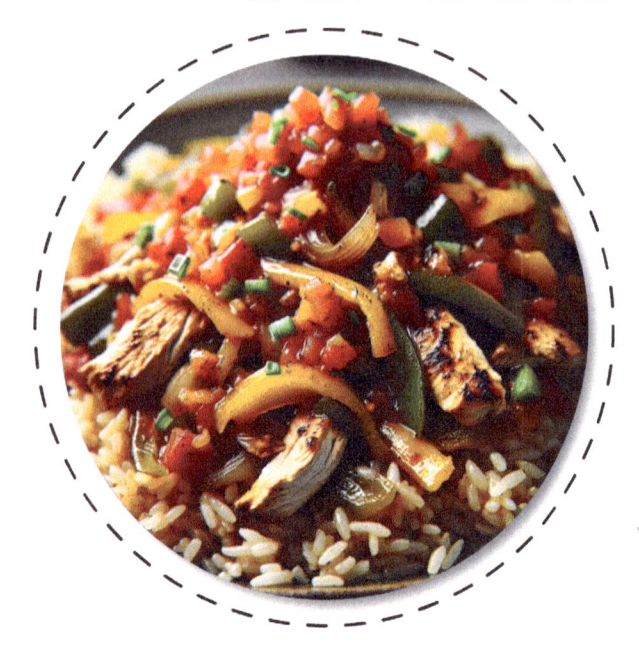

These Chicken Fajita Bowls are a vibrant and satisfying meal packed with classic fajita flavors! Tender, marinated chicken strips are cooked to perfection alongside colorful fajita vegetables. Piled high over nutty brown rice and finished with your favorite toppings like salsa, guacamole, and a dollop of Greek yogurt, it's a healthy and delicious twist on a Mexican favorite.

NUTRITIONAL FACTS *(per serving)*

Calories: 450
Carbohydrates: 50 g
Fiber: 8 g
Protein: 35 g
Fat: 15 g
Sugar: 8 g

INGREDIENTS

For the Chicken and Vegetables

- 1 pound boneless, skinless chicken breasts, sliced into thin strips
- 1 tablespoon olive oil
- 1 tablespoon fajita seasoning (store-bought, or use a combination of chili powder, cumin, paprika, garlic powder, onion powder, salt, and pepper)
- 1 large bell pepper (any color), sliced
- 1 large onion, sliced
- 1 teaspoon lime juice

For Serving

- 2 cups cooked brown rice
- Toppings: salsa, guacamole, Greek yogurt (or sour cream), shredded cheese, chopped cilantro, hot sauce

INSTRUCTIONS

1. In a bowl, combine the sliced chicken, olive oil, and fajita seasoning. Mix well and let marinate for at least 30 minutes or up to several hours in the refrigerator for deeper flavor.

2. Heat a large skillet over medium-high heat. Add the sliced bell peppers and onions, cooking for 5-7 minutes, or until softened and slightly charred. Remove the vegetables from the pan and set aside.

3. In the same skillet, cook the marinated chicken strips for 3-5 minutes per side, or until cooked through and the juices run clear.

4. Return the sautéed vegetables to the pan with the cooked chicken. Squeeze fresh lime juice over the mixture.

5. Divide the cooked brown rice among serving bowls. Top with the chicken and fajita vegetable mixture. Add your choice of toppings like salsa, guacamole, Greek yogurt (or sour cream), shredded cheese, chopped cilantro, and hot sauce (optional).

6. Enjoy! Serve immediately while it's hot!

MUSHROOM & BLACK RICE RISOTTO

SERVES: 2-3 • PREP TIME: 10 MIN • COOK TIME: 40-45 MIN

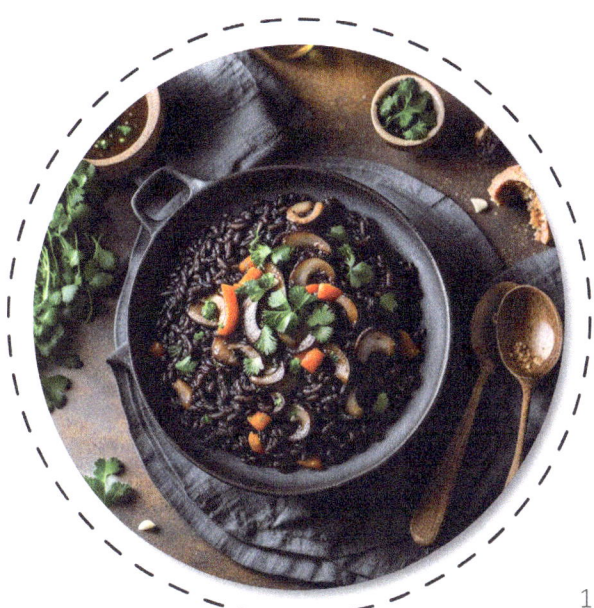

This Mushroom & Black Rice Risotto is a delicious and nutritious twist on a classic! Whole-grain black rice adds fiber and nutrients, while a medley of mushrooms offers savory flavor. It's a lighter take on risotto, letting the natural flavors shine. Plus, you can customize it with your favorite mushrooms for a truly satisfying meal.

NUTRITIONAL FACTS *(per serving)*

Calories: 400
Carbohydrates: 60 g
Fiber: 5 g
Protein: 15 g
Fat: 12 g
Sugar: 5 g

INGREDIENTS

- 1 cup black rice
- 1 tablespoon olive oil
- 1 medium onion, finely chopped
- 2 cloves garlic, minced
- 8 ounces mixed mushrooms (such as cremini, shiitake, oyster), sliced
- 1/2 teaspoon dried thyme
- 1/4 cup dry white wine
- 4-5 cups vegetable broth (warmed)
- 1/4 cup grated Parmesan cheese
- Salt and freshly ground black pepper to taste
- Fresh parsley for garnish (optional)

INSTRUCTIONS

1. Rinse the rice: Rinse the black rice thoroughly in a fine-mesh strainer under cold water.

2. Sauté aromatics: Heat olive oil in a large saucepan or Dutch oven over medium heat. Add onion and cook until softened, about 5 minutes. Add garlic and cook for an additional minute until fragrant.

3. Cook the mushrooms: Add the sliced mushrooms and thyme to the pan. Cook, stirring occasionally, until mushrooms are softened and have released their liquid, about 5-7 minutes.

4. Deglaze the pan: Add white wine to the pan and cook, stirring to scrape up any brown bits from the bottom, until the liquid has reduced by half.

5. Cook the rice: Add the rinsed black rice to the pot and stir to coat. Gradually add the warm vegetable broth, about ½ cup at a time. Stir constantly until the liquid has been absorbed before adding the next portion. Continue this process for approximately 30-40 minutes, or until the rice is tender but still has a slight bite to it.

6. Finish and serve: Remove the pan from the heat and stir in the Parmesan cheese with salt and pepper to taste. Garnish with fresh parsley (if desired) and serve immediately.

LEMON HERB CHICKEN & RICE

SERVES: 2-4 • PREP TIME: 15 MIN • COOK TIME: 25-30 MIN

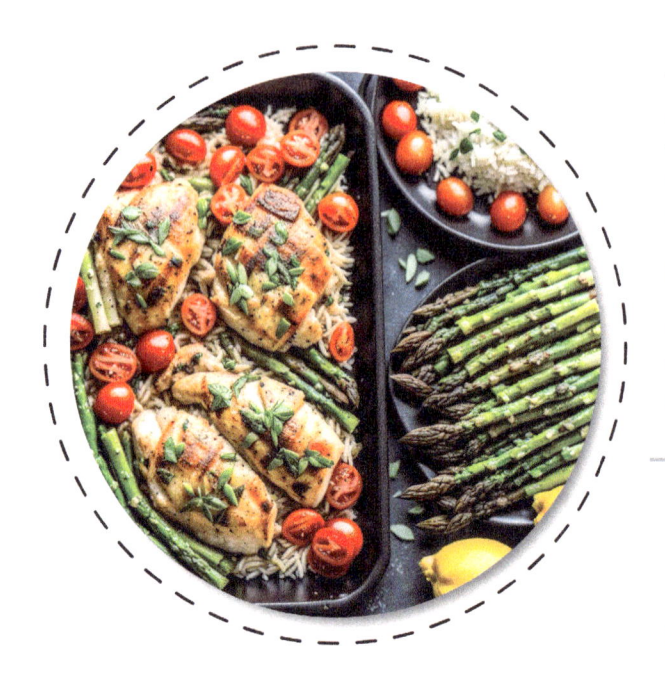

This One-Pan Lemon Herb Chicken & Rice is the perfect healthy and easy weeknight meal! Lean chicken, vibrant asparagus and tomatoes, and fluffy rice cook together in a flavorful broth for maximum nutrition and minimal cleanup. It's a delicious and satisfying meal filled with healthy, whole-food ingredients.

NUTRITIONAL FACTS *(per serving)*

Calories: 450	**Protein**: 35 g
Carbohydrates: 40 g	**Fat**: 15 g
Fiber: 2 g	**Sugar**: 5 g

INGREDIENTS

- 2 bone-in, skin-on chicken breasts (or 4 boneless, skinless chicken thighs)
- 1 tablespoon olive oil
- 1/2 teaspoon dried thyme
- 1/2 teaspoon dried rosemary
- 1/4 teaspoon garlic powder
- Salt and freshly ground black pepper to taste
- 1 cup basmati rice, rinsed
- 1 cup low-sodium chicken broth
- 1/2 cup dry white wine (optional)
- 1 cup chopped asparagus spears
- 1 pint cherry tomatoes
- 1 lemon, sliced
- 4 cloves garlic, peeled

INSTRUCTIONS

1. Preheat your oven to 400°F (200°C).

2. Pat the chicken dry with paper towels. Season generously with olive oil, thyme, rosemary, garlic powder, salt, and pepper.

3. (Optional) Heat a large oven-safe baking dish or skillet over medium heat on the stovetop (if your pan is not oven-safe, you can transfer everything to a baking dish later). Sear the chicken skin-side down for 2-3 minutes, or until golden brown. Flip the chicken and cook for an additional minute.

4. Add the rinsed basmati rice, chicken broth, white wine (if using), chopped asparagus spears, cherry tomatoes, lemon slices, and whole garlic cloves to the baking dish or skillet around the chicken.

5. Cover the pan tightly with a lid (or aluminum foil if your pan doesn't have a lid). Transfer the pan to the preheated oven and bake for 25-30 minutes, or until the rice is cooked through and the chicken is cooked to an internal temperature of 165°F (74°C).

6. Once cooked through, remove the pan from the oven and let it stand for 5 minutes before serving. This allows the juices to redistribute in the chicken for added tenderness. Garnish with fresh herbs like parsley or dill (optional).

CHICKPEA & CAULIFLOWER RICE PILAF

SERVES: 4-6 • PREP TIME: 10 MIN • COOK TIME: 20-25 MIN

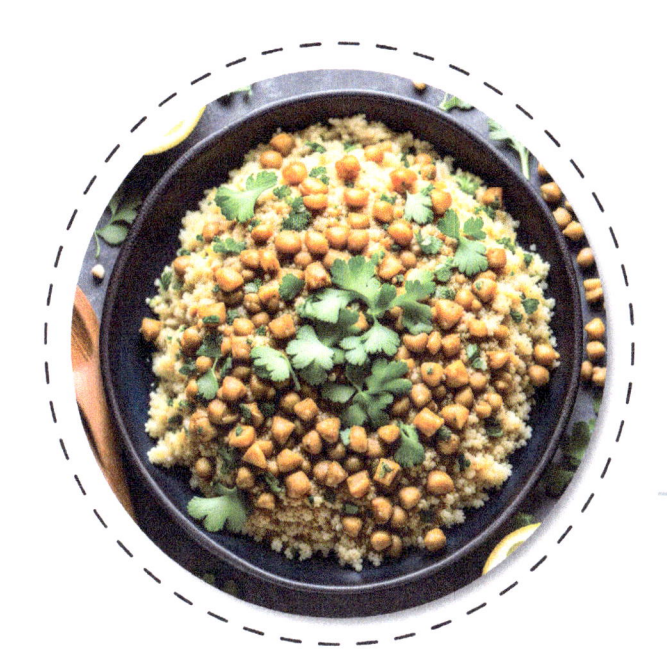

This Cumin-Spiced Chickpea and Cauliflower Rice Pilaf is a flavorful and nourishing plant-based meal! Protein-rich chickpeas and vitamin-packed cauliflower rice combine with warming, anti-inflammatory spices for a dish that's both delicious and good for you. It's an easy and satisfying choice for any night of the week.

NUTRITIONAL FACTS *(per serving)*

Calories: 200
Carbohydrates: 25 g
Fiber: 8 g
Protein: 10 g
Fat: 8 g
Sugar: 5 g

INGREDIENTS

- 1 tablespoon olive oil
- 1 medium onion, chopped
- 2 cloves garlic, minced
- 1 teaspoon ground cumin
- 1/2 teaspoon ground coriander
- 1/4 teaspoon turmeric powder
- 1 (15 ounce) can chickpeas, rinsed and drained
- 4 cups cauliflower rice
- 2 cups vegetable broth (low-sodium preferred)
- 1/4 cup chopped fresh cilantro
- Salt and freshly ground black pepper to taste
- Lemon wedges for serving (optional)

INSTRUCTIONS

1. Heat olive oil in a large skillet or pot over medium heat. Add the chopped onion and cook for 5-7 minutes, or until softened. Add the minced garlic and cook for an additional minute until fragrant.

2. Stir in the ground cumin, coriander, and turmeric powder. Cook for 30 seconds, stirring constantly, allowing the spices to release their aroma.

3. Add the chickpeas and cauliflower rice to the skillet. Stir to combine everything evenly with the spice mixture.

4. Pour in the vegetable broth and bring to a simmer. Reduce heat to low, cover the skillet, and cook for 10-12 minutes, or until the cauliflower rice is tender and most of the liquid has been absorbed.

5. Remove from heat and fluff the cauliflower rice with a fork. Stir in the chopped cilantro and season with salt and pepper to taste. Serve immediately with lemon wedges (optional) for a squeeze of zesty freshness.

LEMON HERB SHRIMP QUINOA SALAD

SERVES: 4 • PREP TIME: 20 MIN • COOK TIME: 10 MIN

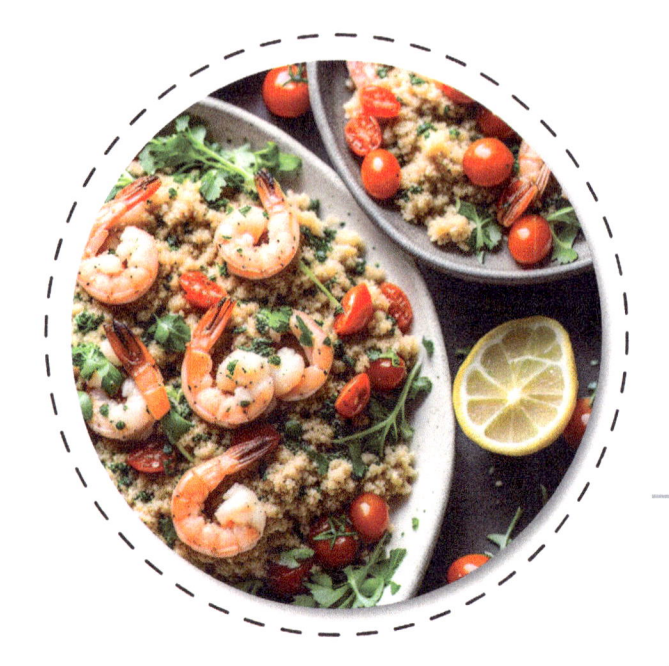

This Lemon Herb Shrimp and Quinoa Salad is a refreshing and healthy meal bursting with flavor! Lean shrimp pairs perfectly with fluffy quinoa for a protein and fiber boost. Cherry tomatoes and arugula add vitamins and antioxidants, while a light lemon herb vinaigrette keeps it bright and delicious.

NUTRITIONAL FACTS *(per serving)*

Calories: 350
Carbohydrates: 25 g
Fiber: 6 g
Protein: 30 g
Fat: 18 g
Sugar: 5 g

INGREDIENTS

For the Shrimp
- 1 pound large shrimp, peeled and deveined
- 2 tablespoons olive oil
- 2 cloves garlic, minced
- 1 tablespoon lemon juice
- 1 teaspoon dried oregano
- 1/2 teaspoon dried thyme
- Salt and freshly ground black pepper to taste

For the Salad
- 1 cup cooked quinoa
- 1 cup cherry tomatoes, halved
- 2 cups arugula
- 1/4 cup chopped fresh parsley

For the Vinaigrette
- 3 tablespoons olive oil
- 2 tablespoons lemon juice
- 1 teaspoon Dijon mustard
- 1 teaspoon honey (optional)
- Salt and freshly ground black pepper to taste

INSTRUCTIONS

1. In a bowl, combine the shrimp, olive oil, garlic, lemon juice, oregano, thyme, salt, and pepper. Toss to coat well and allow to marinate for at least 15 minutes or in the refrigerator for up to 2 hours.

2. **Choose your method**:

   - Grilling: Preheat a grill or grill pan to medium-high heat. Thread the marinated shrimp onto skewers (to prevent falling through the grates) and grill for 2-3 minutes per side, or until pink and cooked through.

   - Sautéing: Heat some olive oil in a pan over medium-high heat. Add the marinated shrimp and cook for 2-3 minutes per side, or until pink and cooked through.

3. Whisk together olive oil, lemon juice, Dijon mustard, honey (optional), salt, and pepper in a small bowl.

4. In a large bowl, combine the cooked quinoa, halved cherry tomatoes, arugula, chopped parsley, and cooked shrimp. Gently toss to mix.

5. Drizzle the vinaigrette over the salad and toss. Season with additional salt and pepper to taste. Serve immediately.

VEGETARIAN THAI PINEAPPLE FRIED RICE

SERVES: 4 • PREP TIME: 15 MIN • COOK TIME: 15-20 MIN

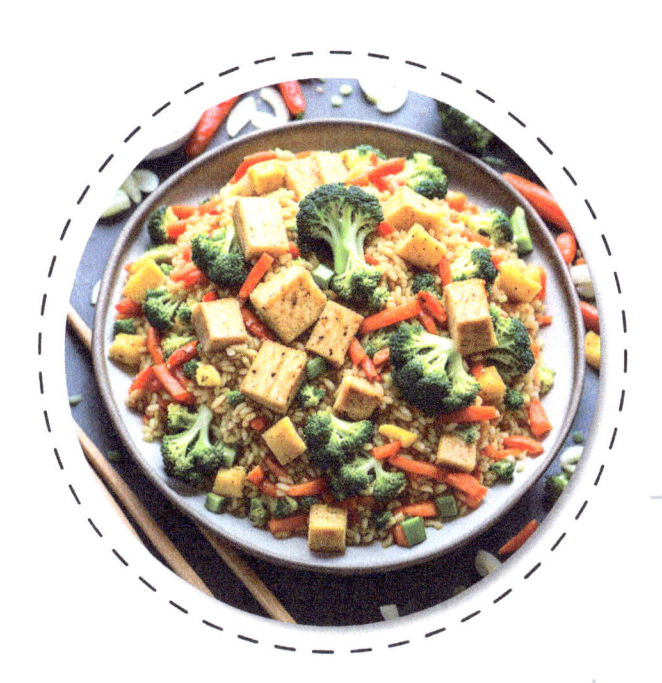

This Vegetarian Thai Pineapple Fried Rice is a healthy and vibrant meal packed with flavor! Tofu delivers plant-based protein, while pineapple and colorful veggies offer a boost of vitamins and antioxidants. It's infused with Thai spices for a sweet, savory, and slightly spicy experience you can customize to your taste.

NUTRITIONAL FACTS *(per serving)*

Calories: 350 **Protein**: 15 g
Carbohydrates: 45 g **Fat**: 15 g
Fiber: 6 g **Sugar**: 15 g

INGREDIENTS

- 1 cup cooked jasmine rice
- 1 tablespoon vegetable oil
- 1/2 block extra-firm tofu, pressed and crumbled
- 1/2 cup chopped onion
- 1 cup mixed vegetables (bell peppers, carrots, broccoli florets, etc.)
- 1 cup diced pineapple
- 2 cloves garlic, minced
- 1 teaspoon Thai curry paste (adjust based on spice preference)
- 2 tablespoons soy sauce (or use low sodium)
- 1 teaspoon sesame oil
- 1/4 cup chopped cashews or peanuts (optional)
- Fresh cilantro for serving (optional)

INSTRUCTIONS

1. If using extra-firm tofu, press it to remove excess moisture. This helps the tofu get crispy when stir-fried. Crumble the tofu into bite-sized pieces.

2. Heat vegetable oil in a large wok or skillet over medium-high heat. Add the crumbled tofu and sauté for 5-7 minutes, or until golden brown and slightly crispy. Remove the tofu from the pan and set aside.

3. Add a little more oil to the pan if needed. Sauté the chopped onion, mixed vegetables, and pineapple for 3-5 minutes, or until the vegetables are crisp-tender. Add the minced garlic and cook for an additional 30 seconds.

4. Add the Thai curry paste to the pan. Cook for 30 seconds, stirring constantly, allowing the spices to release their aroma. Stir in the soy sauce and sesame oil.

5. Return the cooked tofu to the pan. Add the cooked jasmine rice and gently toss to combine. Cook for a few more minutes, or until heated through.

6. Stir in the chopped cashews or peanuts (optional) for an extra layer of crunch. Serve immediately, garnished with fresh cilantro if desired.

INIDIAN LENTIL CURRY BOWL

SERVES: 4 • PREP TIME: 15 MIN • COOK TIME: 30 MIN

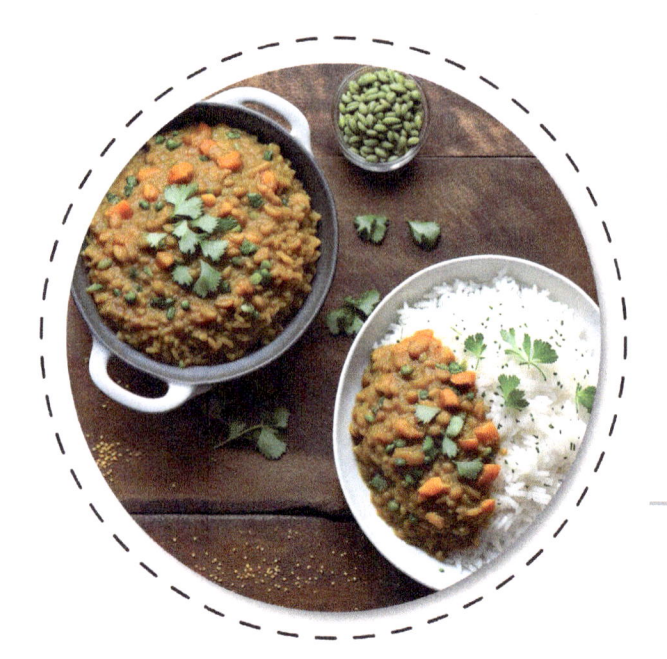

Get ready to transport your taste buds to India with this vibrant and nourishing Indian-Inspired Lentil Curry Bowl! This dish features a fragrant coconut milk-based curry simmered with protein-rich red lentils, vibrant spinach, and a blend of warming spices. Served over a scoop of fluffy basmati rice, it's a satisfying and delicious plant-based meal.

NUTRITIONAL FACTS *(per serving)*

Calories: 400 **Protein**: 18 g
Carbohydrates: 50 g **Fat**: 18 g
Fiber: 12 g **Sugar**: 8 g

INGREDIENTS

- 1 tablespoon olive oil
- 1 medium onion, chopped
- 2 cloves garlic, minced
- 1 tablespoon grated fresh ginger
- 1 teaspoon ground cumin
- 1 teaspoon ground coriander
- 1/2 teaspoon turmeric powder
- 1 (14-ounce) can full-fat coconut milk
- 1 cup vegetable broth
- 1 cup red lentils, rinsed
- 5 ounces baby spinach
- Salt and pepper to taste
- 1 cup cooked basmati rice

INSTRUCTIONS

1. Heat olive oil in a large pot or Dutch oven over medium heat. Add chopped onion and sauté for 5-7 minutes, or until softened. Stir in the minced garlic and grated ginger, cook for 1 minute more, until fragrant.

2. Add cumin, coriander, and turmeric to the pot. Cook for 30 seconds, stirring constantly, allowing the spices to release their aroma.

3. Pour in coconut milk and vegetable broth. Add rinsed red lentils. Bring to a gentle simmer.

4. Reduce heat to low, cover, and simmer for 15-20 minutes, or until lentils are tender and the curry thickens slightly. Stir occasionally to prevent sticking.

5. Add baby spinach to the pot and stir until it wilts. Season generously with salt and pepper to taste.

6. Assemble and enjoy: Divide cooked basmati rice into bowls. Top with a generous scoop of the lentil curry. Serve immediately.

GREEK CHICKEN SKEWERS WITH BROWN RICE

SERVES: 4 • PREP TIME: 30 MIN • COOK TIME: 50 MIN

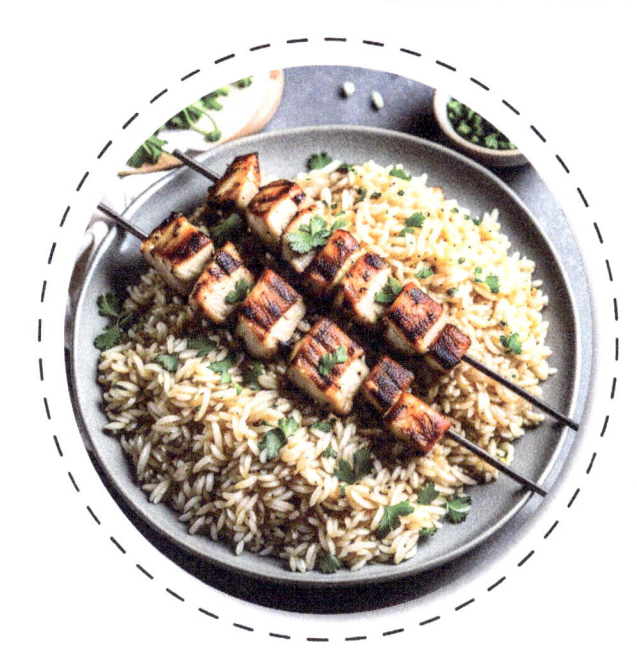

Escape to Greece with these flavorful Greek Chicken Skewers! Juicy chicken, marinated in lemon, olive oil, oregano, and garlic, delivers lean protein and vibrant flavor. Enjoy it with satisfying brown rice pilaf, and cooling tzatziki. This dish is a delicious and healthy way to enjoy a taste of the Mediterranean.

NUTRITIONAL FACTS *(per serving)*

Calories: 600   **Protein**: 40 g

Carbohydrates: 60 g   **Fat**: 25 g

Fiber: 8 g   **Sugar**: 8 g

INGREDIENTS

For the Chicken Skewers

- 1 pound boneless, skinless chicken breasts, cut into 1-inch cubes
- 1/4 cup olive oil
- 2 tablespoons fresh lemon juice
- 1 tablespoon dried oregano
- 1 teaspoon garlic powder
- 1/2 teaspoon dried thyme
- Salt and black pepper to taste
- 12 wooden skewers (soaked in water for at least 30 minutes to prevent burning)

For the Brown Rice Pilaf

- 1 cup brown rice, rinsed
- 1 1/2 cups vegetable broth
- 1 tablespoon olive oil
- 1/2 onion, chopped
- 1/4 cup chopped fresh parsley

INSTRUCTIONS

1. Marinate the Chicken: In a large bowl, combine olive oil, lemon juice, oregano, garlic powder, thyme, salt, and pepper. Whisk well to create a marinade. Add the chicken cubes to the marinade and toss to coat evenly. Cover and refrigerate for at least 30 minutes, or up to 4 hours for deeper flavor.

2. Heat olive oil in a medium saucepan over medium heat. Add the chopped onion and cook for 3-5 minutes, or until softened.

3. Stir in the rinsed brown rice and cook for 1 minute, allowing the rice to toast slightly.

4. Pour in the vegetable broth and bring to a boil. Reduce heat to low, cover the pot, and simmer for 40-45 minutes, or until the rice is cooked through and all liquid is absorbed. Fluff the rice with a fork and set aside.

5. Preheat your grill to medium-high heat. Thread the marinated chicken cubes onto the soaked wooden skewers. Grill the chicken skewers for 8-10 minutes per side, or until cooked through and the juices run clear.

6. Serve and Enjoy! Plate the cooked brown rice pilaf. Top with grilled chicken skewers. Serve with a side of tzatziki sauce and the Greek salad (if using).

MEXICAN CHICKEN & RICE STUFFED PEPPERS

SERVES: 4 • PREP TIME: 20 MIN • COOK TIME: 35 MIN

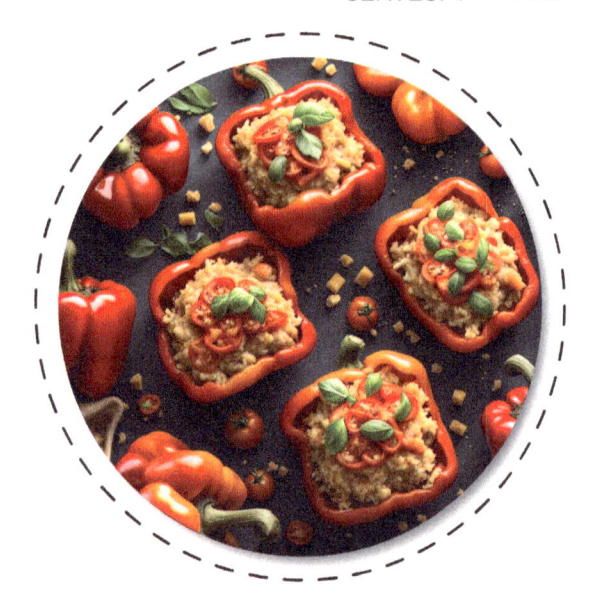

These Mexican Chicken & Rice Stuffed Peppers are a delicious and healthy way to spice up dinnertime! They deliver a balanced mix of protein, complex carbs, and veggies with bold Mexican flavors. The bell peppers act as edible bowls for perfect portion control, and you can easily customize them with your favorite fillings and spice levels.

NUTRITIONAL FACTS *(per serving)*

Calories: 400
Carbohydrates: 30 g
Fiber: 6 g
Protein: 30 g
Fat: 18 g
Sugar: 8 g

INGREDIENTS

- 4 medium bell peppers (any color)
- 1 tablespoon olive oil
- 1 pound ground chicken
- 1/2 onion, chopped
- 1 cup cooked brown rice
- 1 cup frozen or canned corn (drained)
- 1 (14.5-ounce) can diced tomatoes, undrained
- 1 teaspoon chili powder
- 1/2 teaspoon cumin
- 1/2 teaspoon garlic powder
- Salt and pepper to taste
- 1/2 cup shredded Mexican-style cheese blend

INSTRUCTIONS

1. Slice the tops off the bell peppers and remove the seeds and ribs. Try to keep the peppers intact for stuffing.

2. Heat olive oil in a large skillet over medium-high heat. Add ground chicken and cook, breaking it up with a spoon, until browned on all sides.

3. Sauté the onion: Add chopped onion to the skillet with the chicken. Sauté for 3-5 minutes, or until softened.

4. Stir in cooked brown rice, corn, undrained diced tomatoes, chili powder, cumin, garlic powder, salt, and pepper to the skillet.

5. Bring to a simmer, then reduce heat to low and simmer for 5-10 minutes, or until flavors meld and the mixture thickens slightly.

6. Preheat oven to 375°F (190°C).

7. Spoon the chicken and rice mixture evenly into the prepared bell peppers. Top with shredded cheese. Bake for 20-25 minutes, or until cheese is melted and bubbly, and the peppers are tender-crisp.

8. Serve hot, garnished with additional cilantro, green onions, or avocado slices (optional).

INDEX OF RECIPES

BREAKFAST

APPLE-CINNAMON RICE BAKE, p. 24
BANANA-NUT RICE PANCAKES, p. 28
BERRYLICIOUS RICE PUDDING PARFAITS, p.21
FRUITY RICE SALAD, p.29
HUMMUS & VEGGIE RICE WRAPS, p.26
MEDITERRANEAN SCRAMBLE, p.19
PEANUT BUTTER POWER BOWL, p.25
PROTEIN-PACKED FRIED RICE, p.23
SAVORY RICE OMELET, p.20
SOUTHWEST SUNRISE BOWL, p.22
SWEET POTATO RICE PUDDING CUPS, p.27
TROPICAL COCONUT RICE PORRIDGE, p.18
TURMERIC GOLDEN MILK RICE PUDDING, p.30

LUNCH

ASIAN STRI-FRY DELIGHT, p.32
CALIFORNIA-STYLE SUSHI ROLL, p.35
LEMONY SHRIMP & WILD RICE, p.37
MANGO SALSA RICE BOWL, p.40
MEDITERRANEAN WILD RICE BOWL, p.33
SPANISH-STYLE PAELLA, p.41
SPICY BLACK BEAN BURRITO BOWL, p.34
THAI RED CURRY CHICKEN BOWL, p.36
TUSCAN BROWN RICE & LENTIL SOUP, p.39
VIETNAMESE RICE PAPER ROLLS, p.38

SNACKS

CHINESE RED RICE "POPCORN", p.50
CRISPY WILD RICE CRACKERS, p.43
ITALIAN RICE PUDDING PARFAIT, p.51
KOREAN KIMCHI RICE CAKES, p.48
MEDITERRANEAN-INSPIRED RICE BALLS, p.44
PEANUT BUTTER BANANA RICE BITES, p.53
SAVORY SUSHI MUFFINS, p. 46
SPICED BLACK RICE CRACKERS, p.52
SWEET & SALTY BLACK RICE MIX, p.47
THAI COCONUT RICE PUDDING BITES, p.45
TROPICAL FRUIT & RICE SALAD CUPS, p.49

DINNER

CHICKEN FAJITA BOWL, p.56
CHICKPEA AND CAULIFLOWER RICE PILAF, p.59
GREEK CHICKEN SKEWERS WITH BROWN RICE, p.63
INDIAN-INSPIRED LENTIL CURRY BOWL, p.62
LEMON HERB SHRIMP QUINOA SALAD, p.58
MEXICAN CHICKEN & RICE STUFFED PEPPERS, p.64
MUSHROOM & BLACK RICE RISOTTO, p.57
ONE-PAN LEMON HERB CHICKEN & RICE, p.58
SPANISH PAELLA REMIX, p.55
VEGETARIAN THAI PINEAPPLE FRIED RICE, p.61

28-Day Meal Planner

DAY 1

BREAKFAST	TROPICAL COCONUT RICE PORRIDGE, **p.18**
LUNCH	ASIAN STIR-FRY DELIGHT, **p.32**
DINNER	CHICKEN FAJITA BOWL, **p. 56**
SNACKS	KOREAN KIMCHI RICE CAKES, **p. 48**

DAY 2

BREAKFAST	PEANUT BUTTER POWER BOWL, **p.25**
LUNCH	SPICY BLACK BEAN BURRITO BOWL, **p.34**
DINNER	LEMON HERB SHRIMP QUINOA BOWL, **p.58**
SNACKS	CHINESE RED RICE "POPCORN", **p.50**

DAY 3

BREAKFAST	MEDITERRANEAN SCRAMBLE, **p.19**
LUNCH	LEMONY SHRIMP & WILD RICE, **p.37**
DINNER	MUSHROOM & BLACK RICE RISOTTO, **p.57**
SNACKS	TROPICAL FRUIT & RICE SALAD CUPS, **p.49**

DAY 4

BREAKFAST	SAVORY RICE OMELETTE, **p.20**
LUNCH	THAI RED CURRY CHICKEN BOWL, **p.36**
DINNER	SPANISH PAELLA REMIX, **p.55**
SNACKS	SAVORY SUSHI MUFFINS, **p.46**

DAY 5

BREAKFAST	BERRYLICIOUS RICE PUDDING PARFAIT, **p.21**
LUNCH	MEDITERRANEAN WILD RICE BOWL, **p.33**
DINNER	CHICKPEA & CAULIFLOWER RICE PILAF , **p.59**
SNACKS	SWEET & SALTY BLACK RICE MIX, **p.47**

DAY 6

BREAKFAST	SOUTHWEST SUNRISE BOWL, **p.22**
LUNCH	TUSCAN BROWN RICE & LENTIL SOUP, **p.39**
DINNER	MEXICAN CHICKEN & RICE STUFFED PEPPERS, **p.64**
SNACKS	CRISPY WILD RICE CRACKERS, **p.43**

28-Day Meal Planner

DAY 7

BREAKFAST	FRUITY RICE SALAD, **p.29**
LUNCH	SPANISH-STYLE PAELLA, **p.41**
DINNER	GREEK CHICKEN SKEWERS WITH BROWN RICE, **p. 63**
SNACKS	ITALIAN RICE PUDDING PARFAIT, **p. 51**

DAY 8

BREAKFAST	BANANA-NUT RICE PANCAKES, **p.28**
LUNCH	MANGO SALSA RICE BOWL, **p.40**
DINNER	VEGETARIAN THAI PINEAPPLE FRIED RICE, **p.61**
SNACKS	PEANUT BUTTER BANANA RICE BITES, **p.53**

DAY 9

BREAKFAST	APPLE CINNAMON RICE BAKE, **p.24**
LUNCH	VIETNAMESE RICE PAPER ROLLS, **p.38**
DINNER	INDIAN-INSPIRED LENTIL CURRY BOWL, **p.62**
SNACKS	MEDITERRANEAN-INSPIRED RICE BALLS, **p.44**

DAY 10

BREAKFAST	HUMMUS & VEGGIE RICE WRAPS, **p.26**
LUNCH	LEMONY SHRIMP & WILD RICE , **p.37**
DINNER	SPANISH PAELLA REMIX, **p.55**
SNACKS	THAI COCONUT RICE PUDDING BITES , **p.45**

DAY 11

BREAKFAST	SAVORY RICE OMELET, **p.20**
LUNCH	SPICY BLACK BEAN BURRITO BOWL, **p.34**
DINNER	ONE-PAN LEMON HERB CHICKEN & RICE , **p.59**
SNACKS	CHINESE RED RICE "POPCORN", **p.50**

DAY 12

BREAKFAST	PEANUT BUTTER POWER BOWL, **p.25**
LUNCH	THAI RED CURRY CHICKEN BOWL, **p.36**
DINNER	LEMON HERB SHRIMP QUINOA SALAD, **p.58**
SNACKS	SAVORY SUSHI MUFFINS, **p.46**

28-Day Meal Planner

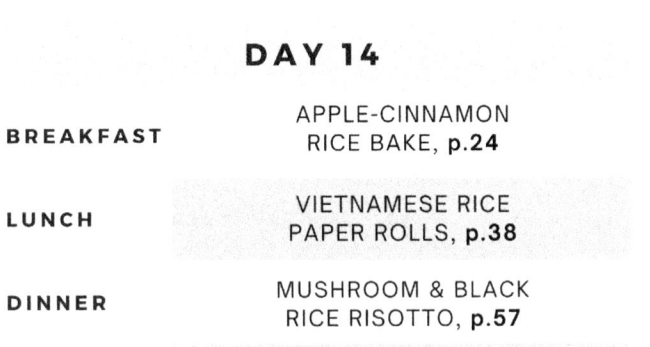

DAY 13

- **BREAKFAST**: SOUTHWEST SUNRISE BOWL, p.22
- **LUNCH**: SPANISH-STYLE PAELLA, p.41
- **DINNER**: CHICKPEA & CAULIFLOWER RICE PILAF, p. 59
- **SNACKS**: KOREAN KIMCHI RICE CAKES, p. 48

DAY 14

- **BREAKFAST**: APPLE-CINNAMON RICE BAKE, p.24
- **LUNCH**: VIETNAMESE RICE PAPER ROLLS, p.38
- **DINNER**: MUSHROOM & BLACK RICE RISOTTO, p.57
- **SNACKS**: TROPICAL FRUIT AND RICE SALAD CUPS, p.49

DAY 15

- **BREAKFAST**: SWEET POTATO RICE PUDDING CUPS, p.27
- **LUNCH**: CALIFORNIA-STYLE SUSHI ROLLS, p.35
- **DINNER**: INDIAN-INSPIRED LENTIL CURRY BOWL, p.62
- **SNACKS**: MEDITERRANEAN-INSPIRED RICE BALLS, p.44

DAY 16

- **BREAKFAST**: TROPICAL COCONUT RICE PORRIDGE, p.18
- **LUNCH**: TUSCAN BROWN RICE & LENTIL SOUP, p.39
- **DINNER**: MEXICAN CHICKEN & RICE STUFFED PEPPERS, p.64
- **SNACKS**: SWEET & SALTY BLACK RICE MIX, p.45

DAY 17

- **BREAKFAST**: BERRYLICIOUS RICE PUDDING PARFAIT, p.21
- **LUNCH**: ASIAN STIR-FRY DELIGHT, p.34
- **DINNER**: VEGETARIAN THAI PINEAPPLE FRIED RICE, p.59
- **SNACKS**: SPICED BLACK RICE CRACKERS, p.50

DAY 18

- **BREAKFAST**: TURMERIC GOLDEN MILK RICE PUDDING, p.30
- **LUNCH**: MEDITERRANEAN WILD RICE BOWL, p.33
- **DINNER**: GREEK CHICKEN SKEWERS WITH BROWN RICE, p.63
- **SNACKS**: THAI COCONUT RICE PUDDING BITES, p.45

28-Day Meal Planner

DAY 19

BREAKFAST	TROPICAL COCONUT RICE PORRIDGE, **p.18**
LUNCH	ASIAN STIR-FRY DELIGHT, **p.32**
DINNER	CHICKEN FAJITA BOWL, **p. 56**
SNACKS	KOREAN KIMCHI RICE CAKES, **p. 48**

DAY 20

BREAKFAST	PEANUT BUTTER POWER BOWL, **p.25**
LUNCH	SPICY BLACK BEAN BURRITO BOWL, **p.34**
DINNER	LEMON HERB SHRIMP QUINOA BOWL, **p.58**
SNACKS	CHINESE RED RICE "POPCORN", **p.50**

DAY 21

BREAKFAST	MEDITERRANEAN SCRAMBLE, **p.19**
LUNCH	LEMONY SHRIMP & WILD RICE, **p.37**
DINNER	MUSHROOM & BLACK RICE RISOTTO, **p.57**
SNACKS	TROPICAL FRUIT & RICE SALAD CUPS, **p.49**

DAY 22

BREAKFAST	SAVORY RICE OMELETTE, **p.20**
LUNCH	THAI RED CURRY CHICKEN BOWL, **p.36**
DINNER	SPANISH PAELLA REMIX, **p.55**
SNACKS	SAVORY SUSHI MUFFINS, **p.46**

DAY 23

BREAKFAST	BERRYLICIOUS RICE PUDDING PARFAIT, **p.21**
LUNCH	MEDITERRANEAN WILD RICE BOWL, **p.33**
DINNER	CHICKPEA & CAULIFLOWER RICE PILAF , **p.59**
SNACKS	SWEET & SALTY BLACK RICE MIX, **p.47**

DAY 24

BREAKFAST	SOUTHWEST SUNRISE BOWL, **p.22**
LUNCH	TUSCAN BROWN RICE & LENTIL SOUP, **p.39**
DINNER	MEXICAN CHICKEN & RICE STUFFED PEPPERS, **p.64**
SNACKS	CRISPY WILD RICE CRACKERS, **p.43**

28-Day Meal Planner

DAY 25

BREAKFAST	FRUITY RICE SALAD, **p.29**
LUNCH	SPANISH-STYLE PAELLA, **p.41**
DINNER	GREEK CHICKEN SKEWERS WITH BROWN RICE, **p. 63**
SNACKS	ITALIAN RICE PUDDING PARFAIT, **p. 51**

DAY 26

BREAKFAST	BANANA-NUT RICE PANCAKES, **p.28**
LUNCH	MANGO SALSA RICE BOWL, **p.40**
DINNER	VEGETARIAN THAI PINEAPPLE FRIED RICE, **p.61**
SNACKS	PEANUT BUTTER BANANA RICE BITES, **p.53**

DAY 27

BREAKFAST	APPLE CINNAMON RICE BAKE, **p.24**
LUNCH	VIETNAMESE RICE PAPER ROLLS, **p.38**
DINNER	INDIAN-INSPIRED LENTIL CURRY BOWL, **p.62**
SNACKS	MEDITERRANEAN-INSPIRED RICE BALLS, **p.44**

DAY 28

BREAKFAST	HUMMUS & VEGGIE RICE WRAPS, **p.26**
LUNCH	LEMONY SHRIMP & WILD RICE , **p.37**
DINNER	SPANISH PAELLA REMIX, **p.55**
SNACKS	THAI COCONUT RICE PUDDING BITES , **p.45**

Printed in Great Britain
by Amazon